T0214560

Clinical Research

John G. Brock-Utne

Clinical Research

Case Studies of Successes and Failures

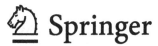 Springer

John G. Brock-Utne
Professor
Department of Anesthesia
Stanford University
Stanford, CA, USA

ISBN 978-1-4939-2515-5   ISBN 978-1-4939-2516-2   (eBook)
DOI 10.1007/978-1-4939-2516-2

Library of Congress Control Number: 2015938594

Springer New York Heidelberg Dordrecht London

Printed on acid-free paper

Springer Science+Business Media LLC New York is part of Springer Science+Business Media (www.springer.com)

For the next generation:
  Matthew B. Brock-Utne
  Tobias J. Brock-Utne
  Anders C. Brock-Utne
  Jasper L. Brock-Utne
  Stefan S. Brock-Utne
  Charlotte E. Brock-Utne

Preface

The intention of this book is to highlight the many pitfalls that can occur when contemplating doing clinical research. This is based on my over 45 years of involvement in clinical research in four continents. Even though some of my mishaps have occurred over 40 years ago, I can assure you that these mistakes occur even to this day with monotonous regularity. Hence the book.

After each case history a question is posed. These are questions you may be faced with as a clinical researcher. The solutions suggested may be controversial and as such may form the basis for discussions on how best to proceed in your special circumstance.

The object of these many stories is to alert the clinical researcher and especially the El Toro researcher that there are many potential disasters waiting to happen when you embark on clinical research. But most of all the reader will hopefully understand that meticulous planning is essential for being successful in this field.

Always remember that the object is to achieve one's research goals quickly with a minimal risk of wasting time and resources.

To quote Marks (1) and to paraphrase Hippocrates of Kos (2):

(1. "The success of research project depends on how well thought out a project is and how potential problems have been identified and resolved before date collection begins" (Marks RG. Designing a research project. The basics of biomedical research methodology. Belmont: Lifetime Learning Publications: A division of Wadsworth 1982).
2. The Art is long
   Life is short
   Experiments perilous
   Decisions difficult.)

Stanford, CA, USA   John G. Brock-Utne

Acknowledgment

To the following, who started me on my clinical research venture. They are presented in the order in which I met them:

1971, Dr. Jon Gjessing, Professor of Anesthesia, Rikshospitalet, University of Oslo, Norway

1973, Dr. John W. Downing, Professor of Anesthesia, University of Natal, Durban, South Africa

1977, Dr. Jay B. Brodsky, Professor of Anesthesia, Anesthesiology, Perioperative and Pain Medicine, Director of the Operating Room at Stanford University School of Medicine, Stanford, CA 94305, USA

A person who must not go unmentioned is my friend Dr. Steve Shafer, Professor of Anesthesiology, Perioperative and Pain Medicine, Stanford University School of Medicine Stanford, CA 94305, USA, and Editor in Chief of *Anesthesia & Analgesia*. His many excellent Editorials and comments about clinical research have been invaluable to me. This is especially true about plagiarism and fraud in clinical research.

To my wife, Sue (48 years married), for her constant encouragement and help with proofreading.

To Shelley Reinhardt (Springer) and Joanna Perey (Springer) for all their help and support

I am also indebted to my research colleagues around the world with whom I have published. I thank them for their hard work, camaraderie, and commitment in our quest to find answers to the questions posed or the clinical observations made. The list is shown below. It may be that I have unintentionally left a few out for which I sincerely apologize.

Barry Adam, Miriam Adhikari, Scott Ahlbrand, Neetu Ahluwalia, John Atchison, Craig T. Albanese, DM Alexander, Karim Ali, Russell Allen, Eric Amador, Gabriel Amir, Nick Anast, Wayne Anderson, Andrew Andrews, Trevor Andrews, Tim Angelotti, Martin Angst, John Archer, Kayvan Ariani, Christopher Arkind, Dave Armstrong, Dan Azar, Nasima Badsha, Brian Baker, Andy J. Barclay, John

J. Barry, John Bean, Peter Bean, David Benaron, Melissa Berhow, Orr Bernstein, Tess Bhatia, Kevin Blaine, Gordon Blake, Paul Blignaut, Patrick Bolton, Gail Boltz, Jerry Bortz, Adrian Bosenberg, Erin Botha, Gregory Botz, Robin Boulle, Jonathan Bradley, Ioana Brisc, Arne J. Brock-Utne, Jay B. Brodsky, Helen M. Bronte-Stewart, Michael Brook, Christopher Brouckaert, Colin Brown, Douglas Brown, Davie Browne, Susan Browne, Carlos Brun, John Bryer, Robert Buley, Ross Bullock, Erin Bushell, Sharon Bux, Jorge Caballero, Pat Callander, Walter Cannon, Alice Cantwell, Brian Cantwell, Carol Canup, Barbara Carr, Brendan Carvalho, Jane Ceranski, Anant Chandel, Peter Chang, Steven D. Chang, Paul Chard, Michael Charles, Robert Cheetham, Marianne Chen, Samuel Chen, Alan Cheng, Rena Chhokra, Alexander Chiu, John Chow, Anne Chowet, Larry F. Chu, Sam Chun, Christopher Church, Rebecca Claure, Michael Coady, Michael Cochran, Sheila Cohen, Anthony Coleman, Jeremy S. Collins, Joe Conradie, Russell Cooper, Jerry Coovadia, Eric Cornidez, John Cosnett, Doug Crockett, Chris Cuerden, John Cummings, Miram Curet, Charles Debattista, Carol A. Diachun, Friederike Dietz, Michael Dillingham, George Dimopoulos, Tom Dow, Laura Downey, John W. Downing, David Drover, Johan DuPreez, Barry Dyck, Paul Eckinger, Henry Edwards, Joshua Edwards, Talmage Egan, Mark Eggen, Christoph Egger-Halbeis, Arne Martin Eide, Inga Elson, Matthew Eng, Herbert Engelbrecht, Michael Ennis, Roy Esaki, Paul Fairbrother, Gary Fanton, Marie Farstad, Bill Feaster, Larry Feld, Vladimir Firago, Steve Fischer, Jason Fleming, Linda Foppiano, Seth Friedland, Maika Fujiki, Louise Furukawa, David M. Gaba, Ray Gaeta, Stephen L. Gaffin, Kingsuk Ganguly, Premjith Gathiram, Monica Gerstner, Rona Giffard, Jon Gjessing, Mark Gjolaj, Christopher Good, Steven Goodman, Stuart Goodman, Neal Goodwin, Dennis Grahn, Lorentz Gran, Mike Greenberg, Ronald Green-Thompson, Mike Gregory, Steve Griffin, Cosmin Guta, Ali Habibi, Alvin Hackel, Gordon Haddow, Ariff Ahmed Haffejee, Jennifer Hah, Christopher Hamilton, David Hamilton, William A. Hampton, Frank L. Hanley, Leland Hanowell, Edmund John Harris, Kyle Harrison, Natalya Hasan, James Healzer, Craig Heller, Jaimie Henderson, Cathy Heninger, Erin K. Hennessey, Erin Hepworth, Jerome Hester, John Hicks, Jesse Hill, Laureen Hill, Gillian Hilton, Lerner B. Hinshaw, Asher Hirshberg, Shawn Hodge, Robert Holbrook, Allan Hold, Jeffrey P. Holden, Allison Holloway, Jung Hong, Susan Hoopes, Peter Houlton, Steve Howard, William Huizinga, David Humphrey, Paul Husby, Jerry Ingrande, Richard A. Jaffe, Mike James, Mark Jamieson, David Jarvis, Stephanie Jeffrey, Chrystina Jette, Derek G. Jordaan, John Jordaan, Bassam Kadry, Ahmed (Mahmood) Kadwa, Hassan Kadwa, Soromini Kallichurum, Sunder Roopsun Kambaran, Komal Kamra, Norman Kaplan, Jadwiga Katolik, Ralph Katzwinkel, Robert Kaye, Michael Keating, Steve Kelleher, Mary Khaing, Muhammad Fazl-Ur Rahman Khan, Andrew Kim, Tae-Wu Edward Kim, Harry Kingston, Yvonne Koen, Marie Koller, Jiang-T Kong, Ted Kreitzman, R Kremer, Vivek Kulkarni, Joseph Kumm, Erin Lachman, Cathy Lammers, Gary Lau, Kenneth Lau, Nigel Lavies, George Lederhaas, Eugene S. Lee, Jennifer Lee, Phoebe Leith, Harry Lemmens, Jody Leng, Theodore Leng, David C. Levi, Robert Levitan, Geoffrey Lighthall, Per Gustav Lilleaasen, Yuan-Chi Lin, Steven Lipman,

Sanford Littwin, N Lopes, Jaime R. Lopez, Andrew Love, Tom Lund, Joe Luther, Alex Macario, Robin MacGillvray, Bruce MacIver, Rob MacKenzie, Sean Mackey, TA MacPherson, Rajend Maharaj, Nisha Malhotra, Ann Marie Mallat, Kevin Mallott, Emmanuel ("Mannie") Mankowitz, Steve Manos, Steve Mantin, Ed Mariano, Masizane Marivate, Jim B.D. Mark, James Mark, Maurice Mars, Aileen Marszalek, William Mathers, Amitabh Mathur, Parag Mathur, Nasim Mayat, Robin McAravey, Larry McFadden, Ashley Micks, Fred Mihm, Samuel A. Mireles, Jon Miser, Lyle L. Moldawer, Vanessa Moll, Jack Moodley, Linesh Moodley, David Morrell, John Morton, Mike Moshal, Ali Mossa, Ryan Mountjoy, Robert Moynihan, Khobi Msimang, Radha Muthukumarasamy, Rai Naidu, Clint Naiker, Sim Naicker, Robert Negrin, Andy Neice, Vladimir Nekhendzy, Camran Nezhat, John Nguyen, Birgit Niestroj, James Nixon, Andy Norbury, Robert Norman Steve O'Keefe, Eli Ohayon, Christopher Olcott, Matthew Oldroyd, Megan Olejniczak, Brent Oskarssen, Einar Ottestad, Ilian Parachikov, David Parris, Andrew Patterson, David Patterson, Nirupa Paulraj, Tim Pavy, Ronald Pearl, Bridget Phillip, Cindy Pillay, Fausto Pinto, John Pollard, Diane Pond, John Propst, Dennis Pudifin, Alex Quick, Deshandra Raidoo, Chandra Ramamoorthy, RJ Ramamurthi, George Ramjee, SA Ramzi, Emily Ratner, Andrew Rauch, Mahmood Razavi, Vadiyala M. Reddy, Catherine Reid, Ed Riley, Sherman Ripley, Archie Ritchie, Peter Ritchie, Frain Rivera, John Robbs, Joe Roberson, George Roberts, Joseph Robertson, Berklee Robins, RM Robins-Browne, Marnie Robinson, Beaver Robles, Tony Rocke, Ed Ronningen, JL Rosen, Jeanne L. Rosner, Chris Rout, Joe Rubin, Cathy Russo, Tom Ruttman, John Ryu, Lawrence Saidman, Robert Salisbury, Stanley Samuels, Rorbert Sanborn, Frank H. Sarnquist, Sunita Sastry, Amit Saxena, Carolyn Schifftner, Cliff Schmiesing, Ingela Schnittger, HS Schoeman, David Schurman, Robert Schuster, Inga Schwegmann, Soraya Seedat, Lars Segadal, David Seidman, Lori Sheehan, Paul Shuttleworth, Lawrence Siegel, Ruwan Amila Silva, Larry Silver, Vanila Singh, Mark Singleton, Jan Sliwa, David Smith, Roy Soetikno, Ezra Sohar, Hugh Brent Solvason, Ted Sommerville, Shaina Sonobe, Eldar Soreide, David Spain, Jean Marie Spitaels, Gary Steinberg, David Stemple, David Stevenson, Robin Stiebel, Marie Strassburg, Paul Strube, Naiyi Sun, David Sze, John Talavera, James Tan, Chris Tataru, Vivianne Tawfik, Renae Tays, Natacha Telusca, Stephen Ternlund, P Tew, J Thai, Kyu Thin, Shaun Mark Thompson, Sandie R. Thomson, Peter John Tomlin, Rodney Torralva, HS Townsend, James R. Trudell, Kendall Truelsen, Brian Tunink, Scott Tweten, Ankeet D. Udani, James Van Dellen, Johan Van den Ende, Pieter Van der Starre, Jason Varner, William Vaughan, G. Hoosen M. Vawda, Mark Vierra, Terry Vitez, Tracey Vogel, Lindsey Vokach-Brodsky, BJ Vorster, Hendrik J. Vreman, David Walker, Brant Walton, Michael Wang, Rachel Wang, David Waterpaugh, Michelle Wells, Steve Welman, Nigel Welsh, Brian Wessels, Mike Wiggins, Frank Wilkins, Deborah Williams, Ron Williamson, Gail Wilmot, Tim Winning, Russell Kong-Yen, Bernhard Wranne, Troy Wu, Imad Yamout, Steve Yu, Amadeo Zanotti, Karl Zheng, Gail Zisook, Andy Zumaran, Gary Zupfer, and Stephan Zweig.

Contents

Basic Premise

A. Why Is Clinical Research Necessary?

Everything we do as physicians carries a potential hazard. It could be the technique and equipment which we use, or it could be the medication which we give. We use these techniques, etc., to treat our patients, hoping that the benefits will outweigh the potential harm. Our clinical decisions are based on what we are mostly taught by our peers, tradition, and some human and many animal studies. Our experience is limited, so where do we get the knowledge to help us make the best decisions to help each patient? The answer is a properly conducted clinical research.

From the early days of medicine, doctors knew that certain treatments were dangerous. Hippocrates of Kos (born 460 BC and died 370 BC) stated: "Primum non nocere" (First, do no harm) and he also said "Desperate diseases require desperate remedies." I remember as a little boy that my father, a doctor, said: "Vondt skal vondt fordrive," which in Norwegian means: "Pain will get rid of pain." He told me this as he lanced an abscess from my finger, without using local anesthesia. (He did not have any.)

Before 1950, there were no government regulations regarding how clinical research should be performed. Most techniques or treatments were brought to the marketplace with minimal or no clinical studies to prove that they were beneficial or, more importantly, safe.

In September/October 1937, a congressional inquiry led to the beginning of the Food and Drug Administration (FDA) after the 73 deaths in the USA from a drug called "Elixir of Sulfanilame." This Elixir contained a solvent, diethylene glycol, which is toxic.

In France, an organic preparation called Stalinon (1956–1957) contained diethyltin diiodide (15 mg) and linoleic acid (100 mg) per capsule. The adult dose was six capsules a day which was a toxic dose. Two hundred and seventeen persons were severely poisoned by Stalinon, and of those, over 100 died.

Even though each country had an FDA of some sort, it was highly ineffective in controlling what was sold to the public. But all this changed with the Thalidomide

(Contergan) tragedy in 1961. The drug, when used by pregnant patients suffering from heartburn, led to the birth of deformed babies. The public all over the world was outraged. Governments decided that the pharmaceutical industry needed to be tightly regulated. As a result, governments decided that they would in the future:

1. Make sure that adequate clinical pharmacological studies would be done on new drugs prior to their release for general use. These studies should include safety testing (in both animals and humans) and clinical trials.
2. Recognize and publish any adverse effects that may arise after the release of a new drug [1].

Hence, clinical research is necessary to answer the questions:

1. How *good* are our medicines, techniques, and equipment?
2. How *bad* are our medicines, techniques, and equipment?

B. Why Do Physicians Do Clinical Research?

Physicians start doing clinical research for various reasons. Many do it because they have passion for a certain technique, drug treatment, and/or a device. They want to show that their idea is better than everyone else's. These researchers often get "bitten by the bug" and make clinical research their life's work.

Others do research purely to get promoted in the university system. The well-known phrase "Publish or Die" is alive and well in academia. An academician's quality and quantity of research output is an easy way to measure his/her academic achievements.

Some people do research to get acknowledged by their peers and to see their name in "golden lights."

Some people do clinical research because of their clinical expertise. Outside agencies recognize this and pay the researcher to conduct research in their field. This financial support can be large and may even pay for part or whole of their annual salary. In addition to the salary, the outside supporters pay the university for using its facilities (usually 35 % of the grand total). In addition, they also pay for research assistants, laboratory fees, etc. In the USA, the financial support to do a 20-patient study can amount to about $300,000.

The individual reasons for doing clinical research vary tremendously and can be one or a combination of any of the above factors. But most importantly, clinical research can be fascinating, rewarding, and fun.

So has the interest in clinical research increased, decreased, or stayed constant in the last 70 years? Take anesthesia, for example. Feneck et al. [2] have indicated that there appears to be a decline in published anesthetic articles. However, Green and Kumar [3] point out that Feneck et al. only reviewed seven journals. It is interesting to note that the first anesthetic journal, *Anesthesia & Analgesia*, came out in 1921.

By 2005, there were 262 anesthetic specialty journals across the world [4]. In the 10 years from 1995 to 2005, there were 56 new journals [4]. Hence, it is more likely that the actual amount of original manuscripts produced in the field of anesthesia has increased tremendously.

C. What Are the Various Experimental Designs?

1. Case report or case series. Simple and mainly descriptive.
2. Random controlled trials. These are considered the "gold standard."
3. Group comparisons. Here, for example, the groups are selected based on the presence or absence of disease.
4. Cohort studies: These can be prospective or retrospective. The groups are selected based on the presence or absence of exposure to treatment, health risks, etc.

There are several sampling methods like random selection, random allocation, or sequential allocation. The method used must include inclusion and exclusion criteria. Statistical analysis must be appropriate and the results summarized clearly. Graphs must be labeled and easy to comprehend.

D. Ethical Issues on Informed Consent and Recruitment for Clinical Trials

It is imperative to obtain informed consent from any patient/volunteer who you want to study. There are obvious moral, sociologic, and legal reasons [5, 6].

My personal success rate in obtaining informed consent is about 50 %. You may think this is low, but I feel that if the patient is unsure about participating, I immediately tell them not to worry and withdraw my proposal. You should never try to pressure people to participate. Patient autonomy must always be respected. If you sense that they are feeling guilty or fearful by not agreeing to participate in your clinical trial, then it is your job to allay their anxiety.

From time to time, I have had patients who have consented to a clinical trial and asked if they can be placed in a specific study group. I have always denied this request as each person is randomly placed in either group. Most clinical researchers will agree with this action. If the requests were agreed to, the groups would no longer be randomized.

There are authors who recommend pre-randomization [7, 8]. This means that patients are randomized to a treatment group before the patient gives consent. Myles et al. [9] found that there was no recruitment improvement when using a pre-randomization protocol. Since they found no benefit and given the ethical concerns raised [9], they recommend that pre-randomization should no longer be used.

References

1. Becker C. Drug pullout. Massive recall of Vioxx poses logistical problems. Mod Health. 2004;34(42):17.
2. Feneck RO, Natarajan N, Sebastian R, Naughton C. Decline in research publications from the United Kingdom in anesthesia journals from 1997–2006. Anaesthesia. 2008;63:270–5.
3. Green J, Kumar S. Apparent decline in published anaesthetic articles. Anaesthesia. 2008;63:1148.
4. Green J, Kumar S. Apparent decline in published anaesthetic articles. Anaesthesia. 2008;63(10):1148–9. http://www.hcuge.ch/anesthesie/anglais/evidence/journals.htm#list.
5. Beecher HK. Ethics and clinical research. NEJM. 1966;274:1354–60.
6. Zelen M. A new design for randomized clinical trials. NEJM. 1979;300:1242–5.
7. Myles PS, Buckland MR, Cannon GB, Bujor M, Langley M, Breaden A, Salamonsen RF, Davis BB. Comparison of patient-controlled analgesia and conventional analgesia after cardiac surgery. Anaesth Intensive Care. 1994;22:672–8.
8. O'Rourke PP, Crone RK, Vacanti JP, Ware JH, Lillehei CW, Parad RB, Epstein M. Extracorporeal membrane oxygenation and conventional medical therapy in neonates with persistent pulmonary hypertension of newborn: a prospective randomized study. Pediatrics. 1989;84:957–63.
9. Myles PS, Fletcher HE, Cairo S, McRae R, Cooper J, Devonshire D, Hunt JO, Richardson J, Machlin H, Morgan EB, Moloney J, Downey G. Randomized trial of informed consent and recruitment of clinical trials in the immediate perioperative period. Anesthesiology. 1999;91:969–78.

Chapter 1
Case 1: A "Good" Question

Before you start doing clinical research, you must have a question that you want to solve. The question should be of great interest to you and you must have a strong passion to solve it.

Equally important as finding the right question is to be very critical of your own idea. You must consider all the various aspects that can possibly prevent you from completing the study, for example, not having enough time, not having enough patients, etc. If you are unsuccessful in finding any reason why you should not attempt to do the study, then you must pursue it steadfastly.

One of the best areas to pick for your research is the one that relates to your everyday practice in the hope to improve patient care. The improvement in patient care has always been my primary motivation for doing clinical research. You can study patients in a primary care setting, a ward, a specialized treatment (dialysis) or investigational unit (endoscopic suites), an ICU, or operating room. Any idea that can benefit patient care is worthy of investigating. But before you embark on your quest, you must prepare well. This will take much longer than you think. Remember the study must be well designed and executed so that it will be accepted for publication. Broadcasting your results is the final and important sequence of the clinical research process.

Prior to the start of the study, you must check that you have everything you need (enough potential patients, equipment, etc.) to be able to answer the question that you will be posing. If you are planning a randomized controlled trial, it is important that the control arm of the study should reflect present clinical practice. Otherwise, how can you interpret the results of the treatment arm? Also consider which peer-reviewed journal will be interested in your study, because you will want, as I say, to get the results published.

The question should be something like:

How good or how bad are our medicines, techniques, or equipment?

Other studies that are acceptable can elucidate mechanism of action in, for example, pharmacology.

© Springer Science+Business Media New York 2015
J.G. Brock-Utne, *Clinical Research*, DOI 10.1007/978-1-4939-2516-2_1

Having found your question, remember to keep it simple and specific. Also never change the question halfway through the study; this may compromise the ability of the data analysis to reach the correct/useful conclusions. By changing the question halfway, you will most likely have changed or modified your end point. Hence, it is imperative to have the correct question to solve from the very beginning and to stick to it.

Here is an example of a good clinical question that we concluded a few years ago [1]:

Does nitrous oxide (N_2O) cause bowel distention in morbidly obese patients during general anesthesia?

There is controversy in the literature if nitrous oxide (N20) can cause bowel distention or not. This information is important to surgeons as should the bowel be distended, it may be difficult to close the abdomen.

Besides this reason, why do you think this was a good study (at least 8 reasons)?

Answer/Solution

It was a good study since:

1. It was a simple study.
2. One end point. Was the bowel distended or not?
3. Surgeon was "blinded" to N_2O being used or not.
4. We had a lot of morbidly obese cases per week.
5. We had interested and supportive surgeons.
6. It was very easy to get consent from the subjects, as there were minimal risks to the patients.
7. It was easy to get IRB approval.
8. There was controversy in the literature (see Chap. 29).

Discussion

That this turned out to be a good question can be seen from the following facts that are summarized below:

1. July 2004. Defined the question, invited the surgeon to participate as "a blinded observer" to N_2O being used or not, wrote out the proposal, and submitted it to the IRB.
2. September 2004. IRB approval.
3. September 2004. Study started. Fifty patients were enrolled.
4. November 2004. Study finished, stats done, and paper written up and submitted. For your information, a simple t-test, Fisher's exact test, or chi-squared tests were used for intergroup comparisons.
5. December 2004. Four weeks after submission, the paper was accepted for publication.

The question was answered: Surgeons could not differentiate if N_2O was used or not. Therefore, the use of N_2O in these cases is an acceptable practice.

Lesson

To do research, you must have a question. This must be simple and when the study is finished, it should preferably give you a "yes" or a "no" answer.

Reference

1. Brodsky JB, Lemmens HJM, Collins JS, Morton JM, Curet MJ, Brock-Utne JG. Nitrous oxide and laparoscopic bariatric surgery. Obes Surg. 2005;15:494–6.

Chapter 2
Case 2: A "Bad" Question

Many years ago, while working as an anesthesiologist and critical care registrar (resident) in King Edward VIII Hospital, University of KwaZulu-Natal, Durban, South Africa, I got interested in the following question:

Does chest physiotherapy (CPT) have a role in the prevention of postoperative respiratory failure after upper abdominal surgery?

I was young and I thought the question could easily be answered, since some surgeons used CPT postoperatively and some did not prescribe to it. Hence, I had two groups. The IRB was easily obtained and so was the consent. I also knew that there would be no lack of patients because upper abdominal knife wounds were very common at our hospital at that time.

After 30 cases, I reviewed the data sheets with my research nurse. On the basis of these findings, we stopped the study. We had not taken into account the many clinical variables that can affect a result.

What variables do you think they were (at least 8)?

© Springer Science+Business Media New York 2015
J.G. Brock-Utne, *Clinical Research*, DOI 10.1007/978-1-4939-2516-2_2

Answer/Solution

The study was stopped as it had not taken into account the following (in no particular order):

1. Associated injuries/diseases.
2. Length of surgery, due to the surgical problems and surgeon's skills.
3. Smoking history.
4. Frequency and duration of CPT.
5. Different types of CPT by different physiotherapists.
6. Antibiotics. Some surgeons used them and some did not.
7. If the antibiotics were used, the timing and dosing of the antibiotics varied tremendously.
8. Mucolytics/bronchodilators. Some physiotherapists used one or the other or both and some did not use any.

Lesson

Always consider the multiple causes that can change a clinical outcome.

Chapter 3
Case 3: Why Were 116 Patients Excluded?

In Case 2, you learned to always consider the multiple causes that can change a clinical outcome. In the end in Case 2, there were no results to write about. So what would you do when faced with this dilemma? Give up or start again?

We redesigned the study and took into account all the points mentioned in solution made in Case 2. After many months, we reviewed the findings. Two hundred and twelve patients had been enrolled successfully. But we had to exclude a total of 116 patients.

Why were these 116 cases excluded?

© Springer Science+Business Media New York 2015
J.G. Brock-Utne, *Clinical Research*, DOI 10.1007/978-1-4939-2516-2_3

Answer/Solution

The 116 cases were excluded mainly because the surgeons had used different antibiotics from the ones we had agreed to. Furthermore, we found that the antibiotics were not given preoperatively as prescribed.

Other causes of exclusion included the differences in physiotherapy techniques and the duration of the therapy. The physiotherapists had been instructed how to do the therapy and had agreed to do it using a mucolytic. However, when reviewing the data sheet and later when questioning the physiotherapists, some had not adhered to the instructions.

We gave up the study. But I learned many lessons from this disaster. I mention them here for your benefit:

1. Always be aware of the multitude of changes that can alter a clinical result.
2. If you rely on other health-care providers in the treatment, make sure that you invite them to be authors, should the results be publishable. This makes them more accountable.
3. Always routinely check the status of trials by regularly reviewing the data sheet, observe how the physiotherapy is done, make sure the antibiotic is given at the prescribed time, etc.
4. Never let clinical trials go over one year. People involved with the study will get bored, lose focus, cut corners, etc.

The best thing to do in a proposed study that involves many different departments and researchers is to do a trial run. You will not regret it.

Lesson

Make sure you have a simple question. Minimize most/all the clinical changes that can affect your results and conclusion.

Chapter 4
Case 4: Sometimes a Good Question Evolves from a Bad One

Case 2 told you about a "bad" question and what happened. Should this happen to you, then always reflect on the bad outcome.

We decided that the biggest "killer" of this study was that the timing of the antibiotics was *not* adhered to. At the time, there was very little literature on the pharmacokinetics of the potential importance of giving prophylactic antibiotics prior to a surgical incision. There were recommendations that preoperative antibiotics should be given prophylactically prior to abdominal surgery, but there was no scientific proof that this would be beneficial.

What study would you now propose to try and address the lack of pharmacokinetics data?

© Springer Science+Business Media New York 2015
J.G. Brock-Utne, *Clinical Research*, DOI 10.1007/978-1-4939-2516-2_4

Answer/Solution

Since wound sepsis commonly occurs in the subcutaneous fat tissue, we decided to study the pharmacokinetics of a preoperative antibiotic in subcutaneous fat.

Discussion

We proposed a study that had not been done previously. We were optimistic that our results would be published as the answer to our question would be useful to the clinician.

We gave prophylactic parenteral cefuroxime (a cephalosporin derivative) and measured the subcutaneous concentrations in laparotomy wounds. Hence, we designed a study entitled:

"What are the plasma/tissue levels after an antibiotic is given IV prophylactically?"

The study was completed and published [1]. The study concluded that subcutaneous tissue peak levels were reached within 15 min, and the tissue half-life was 1.5 h. Since then, many similar studies have been performed, looking at antibiotics and the risk of surgical site infection [2, 3].

Lesson

If a study you have done proves to be non-publishable, then it is imperative that you evaluate what went wrong. Not only do you learn from your mistakes, but you may find something else that could be worth investigating.

References

1. Huizinga WK, Hirshberg A, Thomson SR, Elson KI, Salisbury RT, Brock-Utne JG. Prophylactic parenteral cefuroxime: subcutaneous concentration in laparotomy wounds. J Hosp Infect. 1989;13:395–8.
2. Barie PS, Eachempati SR. Surgical site infections. Surg Clin North Am. 2005;85:1115–35.
3. Toma O, Suntrup P, Stefanescu A, London A, Mutch M, Kharasch E. Pharmacokinetics and tissue penetration of Cefoxitin in obesity: implications for risk of surgical site infection. Anesth Analg. 2011;113:730–7.

Chapter 5
Case 5: What Went Wrong?

One of my colleagues completed a clinical research study in 1968 entitled:

Is there a difference between maternal and neonatal blood gases comparing epidural versus general anesthesia at delivery from a Cesarean section (C/S)?

This was a very good question in 1968. At that time, 99 % of all C/S in the Western World were done under general anesthesia. Not like it is today [1]. Hence, the study question was current and had not been undertaken previously.

General anesthesia at that time was given in the following routine manner [2]. It is summarized; thus, it consisted of a preoperative stomach tube (emergency only) [3], preoxygenation, rapid sequence induction and intubation with thiopental/etomidate/ketamine and succinylcholine, and cricoid pressure. Maintenance was with N_2O, oxygen, and halothane/ether. Muscle relaxation was either with curare or succinylcholine drip.

After 11 months, 240 patients had been studied. They were divided randomly into two groups. The results showed no difference in the neonatal acid base status between the two anesthetic techniques. Although this was a "negative result," my colleague submitted it for publication, knowing that both negative and positive findings are equally valuable. All the reviewers agreed this was an important study, as it was timely, not studied before, and reassuring to the obstetrical anesthesiologist.

However, no journal was interested in publishing it.

Why were no journals interested?

© Springer Science+Business Media New York 2015
J.G. Brock-Utne, *Clinical Research*, DOI 10.1007/978-1-4939-2516-2_5

Answer/Solution

The reason was that no thorough literature search had been done prior to the study.

Discussion

If a search had been conducted, my colleague would have known that all patients for Cesarean section should have been placed on a pelvic tilt. In his study, no tilt had been placed routinely, except in cases when maternal hypotension was noted while the patient was lying flat. The data sheet did not have a "box" for the presence or absence of a tilt. As mentioned, no journal wanted it and hence no publication came of it, despite all the hard work.

Lesson

1. When you have defined your question, you must attempt to learn as much as you can about the proposed study before you embark on it. You must know the literature that pertains to your research question extremely well.
2. Keep more information on the data sheet than you think is important. More is better.

References

1. Lipman S, Carvalho B, Brock-Utne JG. The demise of general anesthesia in obstetrics: prescription for a cure. Int J Obstet Anesth. 2005;14:2–4.
2. Buley RJR, Brock-Utne JG, Downing JW, Houlton PJC. Anesthesia for caesarean section – an updated review of its special problems and their management. S Afr Med J. 1978;54:525–7.
3. Brock-Utne JG, Rout C, Moodley J, Mayat N. Influence of preoperative gastric aspiration on the volume and pH of gastric contents in obstetric patients undergoing caesarean section. Br J Anaesth. 1989;62:397–401.

Chapter 6
Case 6: Check Your Facts

In the USA, the anesthesia practice is to discard the breathing circuits after their use in one patient. This is opposite to the practice in Europe. Here they do not discard the breathing circuits between patients, but only the anesthesia filter that is situated between the anesthesia machine and the patient breathing circuit.

We asked the following clinical research question:

Does the use of a breathing circuit filter prevent the necessity to discard breathing circuits after one use?

We thought this could be a good idea to attempt to introduce the European practice into the USA. Our main thrust was to reduce the landfill.

We designed a study that would show any evidence of bacteria and/or viruses in the anesthetic breathing circuit after use. The samples for bacteria and virus were taken before the filter, in the filter, and after the filter. Samples from 200 patients used breathing circuits (used one time by each patient) were tested and submitted for analysis for bacteriology and virology. The study cost $20,000 which we paid up front.

Finally when the results were sent to us, they were totally useless as there was evidence of an over 30 % contamination of the samples.

How could this happen?

© Springer Science+Business Media New York 2015   13
J.G. Brock-Utne, *Clinical Research*, DOI 10.1007/978-1-4939-2516-2_6

Answer/Solution

The cause of the contamination lay with the technician

Discussion

The technician had assured us that he knew how to do it. After the results came out we asked him to show us how he did the sampling. We immediately understood our dilemma as his collection technique was seen not to be as prescribed nor did he wash his hands before or after the collection.

Since the study was so expensive, we did not have the resources to repeat it.

Lesson

1. Always check that the one or the ones who are doing the sampling know the correct sampling methodology and are continuously doing the same technique for each sampling.
2. Always check that the methodology is being adhered to, by being present, or arriving unannounced on the scene, from time to time.

Chapter 7
Case 7: All Is Not Lost

The fiasco in Chap. 6 led as mentioned to a large loss of lot of research funds and no publication.

We felt deflated and wondered if there was anything we could do with all our knowledge about the reuse of anesthesia breathing systems.

What would you suggest?

© Springer Science+Business Media New York 2015
J.G. Brock-Utne, *Clinical Research*, DOI 10.1007/978-1-4939-2516-2_7

Answer/Solution

Write an editorial. We did and entitled it:
   The reuse of anesthesia breathing systems: another difference of opinion and practice between the United States and Europe [1].

Discussion

The main reason for the differences in practice is both cultural and medicolegal. Scientifically there would seem to be no reason why a breathing system should not be reused. Certainly this would reduce the landfill.

   In a previous study [2], we concluded that all breathing filters retain moisture in healthy patients undergoing general anesthesia. But there are significant performance differences between the various filters, and the performance may not correspond to the manufacturer's specifications. This difference could of course also occur in relation to viruses and bacteria. Hence more studies are needed if this practice is to be adopted in the USA.

Lesson

If you have done a lot of reading around a topic, even performed a study which does not get published, always consider a "free-standing" editorial. With all your knowledge on a topic, this may prove to be a contribution to the literature.

References

1. Egger Halbeis CB, Macario A, Brock-Utne JG. The reuse of anesthesia breathing systems: another difference of opinion and practice between the U.S. and Europe. J Clin Anesth. 2008;28:81–3.
2. Lemmens HJM, Brock-Utne JG. Heat and moisture exchange devices. Are they doing what they are supposed to do? Anesth Analg. 2004;98:382–5.

Chapter 8
Case 8: An Important Lesson

In 1975 we had collected the largest prospective series in the world (over 40 cases) of the anesthetic management of stabbed hearts. We had successfully anesthetized over 40 cases of stabbed hearts in Durban, South Africa. All patients were stabbed within 30 min to 2 h prior to admission.

The study had taken 4 months. One Friday evening I put all the patients' data sheets into my briefcase to review at home over the weekend. On my way home, I stopped over at the Yacht club and left the briefcase in the car. I guess you can imagine what happened.

My briefcase was stolen from my locked car. All the data sheets were lost. I never found the bag or its contents.

So why were my coworkers and I so upset?

© Springer Science+Business Media New York 2015
J.G. Brock-Utne, *Clinical Research*, DOI 10.1007/978-1-4939-2516-2_8

Answer/Solution

We had not made any copies of the data sheets. Since we never found them and I had no other identifiers as to the patients' name or medical record numbers, we had no results and hence no publication.

Today you would most likely have scanned the data sheets onto the computer. Don't throw away the paper data sheets as I know of a friend who had all his Ph.D. data on his computer, no paper data sheets, and the computer got stolen.

Lesson

Always make copies of patient's date sheets and consent forms. This is especially true if you are transporting the data from one place to another. Also never give a coworker any research data sheets before making copies. Back up your data from your computer.

Chapter 9
Case 9: A Lucky Escape

A patient had consented to a study to assess myocardial wall motion during his hip replacement. A *trans*esophageal echocardiogram (TEE) was to be used. There are two anesthesiologists in the room, one looking after the patient while the other was doing the study. After the patient was anesthetized, the TEE probe was to be inserted into the esophagus by one of the anesthesiologists. The patient was in the left lateral position. The insertion proved difficult and the colleague looking after the patient was asked to help. One anesthesiologist was flexing and pulling the jaw forward while the other was navigating the scope.

What is wrong with this picture?

© Springer Science+Business Media New York 2015
J.G. Brock-Utne, *Clinical Research*, DOI 10.1007/978-1-4939-2516-2_9

Answer/Solution

While they were struggling to place the probe, a third anesthesiologist arrived into the operating room. He looked at the monitors and informed them that the patient's BP was 60/20 mmHg. In their attempt to place the probe, they had forgotten to keep an eye on the patient's vital signs. In this case the BP was quickly restored and the patient did very well.

Someone must be solely responsible for the care of a research subject who is being sedated or given a general anesthetic. The other researcher can then peacefully and with confidence gather clinical information from the sedated/anesthetized subject.

Lesson

A designated health care provider must always be in charge of looking after a research subject, especially if they are sedated/anesthetized. This should be his/her sole job.

Chapter 10
Case 10: A Letter or a Full Paper

We did a laboratory study entitled:

Do autoclaved reusable LMAs contain significant protein contamination?

It was very well received at the ASA annual meeting in 2002 [1]. Three months later we submitted the full manuscript to Anesthesiology. Six weeks later we got a communication from the editor stating that he liked it. However he wanted us to cut it down and submit it as a letter. The editor offered, if we accepted, to have an editorial in the same issue as the letter, highlighting and commenting favorably on our submission.

Left with this offer, what would you do? Accept it or seek publication elsewhere?

© Springer Science+Business Media New York 2015

J.G. Brock-Utne, *Clinical Research*, DOI 10.1007/978-1-4939-2516-2_10

Answer/Solution

We decided that a letter was not what we wanted and decline their offer. This turned out to be a mistake.

Discussion

Instead we decided to enlarge the study by including laryngoscopes to see if they too contained protein contamination. We were hoping that with this addition our submission would be accepted as a full article.

It sounded like a reasonable idea at the time to include the laryngoscopes. However, we had not realized how little enthusiasm there was for completing the study. Six years after the initial presentation of the abstract, we eventually submitted our revised paper. The paper was refused two times in North American anesthesia journals, since by now disposable LMAs have entered the market place. Therefore our results were of very little clinical importance. We eventually got it published in 2008 in a foreign journal as we highlighted the fact that in the developing world nearly all used LMAs are reused. Hence our message was to warn the readership of this potentially dangerous practice [2].

Lesson

If you get an opportunity to publish in a good journal, even as a letter, then it is worth accepting it. This is especially true if there is an accompanied editorial.

Be careful when you decide to enlarge a completed study by asking: "It may be a good idea, but are we really interested/willing in finishing the proposed revised study as it will be more work?"

References

1. Chu LF, Trudell JR, Brock-Utne JG. Autoclaved reusable laryngeal mask airways contain significant protein contamination. Anesthesiology. 2002;96:A570.
2. Chu LF, Mathur PN, Trudell JR, Brock-Utne JG. Contamination problems with reuse of laryngeal mask airways and laryngoscopes. Saudi J Anesthesia. 2008;2:58–61.

Chapter 11
Case 11: This Could Be Serious. Be Prepared

You are an assistant professor in a university hospital, with a special interest in a specific aspect of clinical anesthesia. In this field you have published extensively. A startup company representative meets you and suggests collaboration. They have been developing a prototype machine that could prove very useful and helpful for patient care in the field in which you are an expert. You ask to see their preliminary results but are told that the information could not be shared with you. The company representative suggests that you be principal investigator (PI) on a protocol that they are submitting to various venture groups for funding. The representative tells you that the protocol is already written and must be submitted by the next day. He hands you the front page of the protocol and you see your name as the PI. You reply that you need to see the device plus the full protocol, with the preliminary results, before agreeing to participate. The representative says that this is no problem, leaves, and says he will be in contact. Two weeks go by and you hear nothing.

Should you be concerned that the protocol may have been submitted with your name listed as the PI? If so, what should you do about it?

© Springer Science+Business Media New York 2015
J.G. Brock-Utne, *Clinical Research*, DOI 10.1007/978-1-4939-2516-2_11

Answer/Solution

This happened to a friend of mine. None of his phone calls to the company were returned and there were no responses to his many emails. He sent follow-up emails and a certified letter to the representative with a copy to the CEO of the company. In the letter, he clearly stated that he had not seen the preliminary results, the device, nor the full protocol and that he was concerned that the protocol with his name as a PI may have been sent to venture capitalist seeking funding. In addition, he wrote that he did not want his name associated with the device in any shape or form. But he heard nothing from them (I recommended also that he send a copy of the certified letter to himself. When he got it, he should not open it but leave it in a file with the company's name).

Discussion

Several months later he got a phone call from a person who said he was from a venture capital firm. The person wanted to know about the device as my friend was recorded as the PI. My friend told the story about his interaction with the company and sent him a copy of the emails and letters and offered to show him the certified letter that he had sent the company and himself several months before.

Interestingly my friend never heard from either the company or the venture capital firm again.

Lesson

There are many sharks out there, so do watch out.

Chapter 12
Case 12: Not Correct Procedure

As a favor to a colleague from another department, you read through a draft chapter about nausea and vomiting. The colleague is the editor of a new textbook where this chapter is to be included. The chapter is written by a medical student and needs a lot of work before it is ready for submission. You spend an excessive amount of time rewriting the chapter and making major corrections/suggestions. Then you send it back to the medical student and to your colleague.

You hear nothing from either the editor or the medical student. A year later, without warning, the galley proof of the chapter arrives in the mail. As you know, you typically have 48 h to read your submission and return it.

When you look at the galley proof, you see that you are the second author. You start reading the chapter and realize that this is unacceptable. You find the original submission by the medical student and your corrections and realize quickly that the medical student and editor have ignored ALL your corrections/suggestions.

You communicate immediately with the editor via phone telling him that you do not want your name on this publication. He tells you there is nothing he can do and he needs you as author.

What will you do? Is there anything you can do?

© Springer Science+Business Media New York 2015
J.G. Brock-Utne, *Clinical Research*, DOI 10.1007/978-1-4939-2516-2_12

Answer/Solution

This happened to me. Luckily, as mentioned, I had kept a copy of my corrections, together with the original submission by the student.

I got hold of the publisher and sent him a copy of my corrected version of the chapter.

The publisher replied that he could not make all those corrections to the galley. I then told him that at no point was I informed that I would be an author. I was doing the corrections/suggestions only as a favor to my colleague. Luckily the publisher agreed with me and was kind enough to remove my name from the authors' list.

Lesson

When asked to read/correct/make suggestion to a paper/chapter, always keep copies of everything. It is important to also find out if they are considering including you on the authors' list. If so, then it is imperative that you insist on seeing the final draft. If corrections/suggestions that you have made are not included and you feel strongly about them, then you can inform your coworkers that you do not wish to be an author.

Chapter 13
Case 13: A Lesson Well Learned

Forced air patient warming system such as Bair Hugger (BH) (Augustine Medical Inc., Eden Prairie, MN, USA) is a clinically effective patient warming device. Forced air is entrained through a microbial filter (0.2 μm pore size). The air is heated and blown through a detachable hose. The hose is attached to blankets with perforation on its underside. However a potential disadvantage is that BH may blow contaminated air over the surgical wound [1–4]. It does that by sucking pathogens from the floor and delivering them to the surgical field if the filter is not working or exhausted. The BH can also mobilize the patient skin organisms onto the surgical field. Pathogens from the BH tubing (which has been lying on the floor between cases) can also be delivered to the surgical field.

To test if this really is a problem, we took cotton swabs from the distal end of the BH tubing and filter of the BH in all the operating rooms (ORs) in our hospital. We also placed petri dishes in all ORs.

The study was done at the time when it had been recommended that the BH filters be changed after 6 months or more than 500 h of usage. After the study the filters were discarded and replaced. Three months later the study was repeated again.

A total of 90 dishes were sent to the pathology laboratory and clearly labeled with instructions as to what to do. $5,000 was paid up front to isolate all pathogens.

However there was one instruction that we did not stress strongly enough to the pathology department. What do you think that was?

© Springer Science+Business Media New York 2015
J.G. Brock-Utne, *Clinical Research*, DOI 10.1007/978-1-4939-2516-2_13

Answer/Solution

We did not stress the importance of identifying the individual pathogens.

Discussion

So the only results we got from the laboratory were the presence or the absence of pathogens. There were no more results to be had as all the dishes had been thrown out. Hence we only got an abstract out of all this work [2].

Although the chief of pathology had understood that we wanted the individual pathogens, he had not passed on this information to the laboratory technician who was doing the test.

A further problem was the fact that we were not given access to the pathology department when we came with our samples. An administrative assistant, and not the person that was doing the testing, took the samples from us at the heavily guarded door.

Lesson

When you hand over samples to be analyzed, make sure that you hand them to the person that is doing the work. Make sure that he or she understands what is required. If you can't get in to the laboratory, like in this case, it is imperative to make sure that you somehow contact the person doing the testing. Insist that they repeat the instructions of what is required.

References

1. Avidan MS, Jones N, Khoosal M, Lundgren C, Morrell DF. Convection warmers – not just hot air. Anaesthesia. 1997;52:1073–6.
2. Gjolaj M, Ahlbrand S, Yamout I, Armstrong D, Brock-Utne JG. Don't forget to change the Bair Hugger filter. Am Soc Anesthesiol. 2009; Abstract #1168. 17–21 October New Orleans, LA
3. Bassinet L, Matrat M, Njamkepo E, Aberrane S, Housset B, Guiso N. Nosocomial pertussis outbreak among adult patients and healthcare workers. Infect Cont Hosp Ep. 2004;25: 995–1001.
4. Bernards AT, Harinck HIJ, Diijkshoorn L, Van der Reijden TJK, van den Broek PJ. Persistent Acinetobacter baumannii. Look inside your medical equipment. Infect Cont Hosp Ep. 2004; 25:1002–4.

Chapter 14
Case 14: Taking Out a Patent. Should You or Should You Not?

You have made and perfected a medical device and consider taking out a patent in your name. You have done studies to show that it works favorably compared to similar devices on the market. These studies have not been published. You consult a patent lawyer. He strongly suggests that you consider patenting it. The price tag he quotes you for a worldwide patent is $400,000. You have the money, if you put up securities as collateral.

Should you or should you not follow your patent lawyer's advice?

© Springer Science+Business Media New York 2015   29
J.G. Brock-Utne, *Clinical Research*, DOI 10.1007/978-1-4939-2516-2_14

Answer/Solution

My advice is: Don't do it.

Discussion

Don't take out the patent yourself, unless you are very wealthy. Why? You will lose. It has not only happened to me but to many of my friends.

An example of what can happen, after you have a patent, is the following story:

A colleague of mine had paid, with his own money, to get a medical device produced and was selling it with some success. He was approached by a big medical distribution company who wanted to be the sole seller of the device. This medical company was selling a similar but inferior device, which had been shown not to be as effective as his. The company assured my colleague that they would not be selling their device if he signed the contract. My friend agreed to let them have sole sales for 3 years and signed the contract with a minimal sales target. However, after 1 year, the company had not sold any of his devices and, contrary to the contract, had continued to sell the inferior device. He tried to break the contract, but found it impossible.

At the same time, a manufacturer in a foreign country started to make and sell with great success a copy of my colleague's device, without his permission. The foreign company knew that my colleague did not have the finances to defend his patent.

Lesson

1. Don't pay for a patent yourself unless you are very wealthy.
2. Rather take a patent out with a university or a big organization, you may not get a large percentage but you should get something.

Chapter 15
Case 15: Taking Out a Patent. Watch Out

You have discovered a new piece of medical equipment while working at the university. The university is very excited and obtains a worldwide patent for your equipment. The usual arrangement is that you will get about 15–33 % of the income from the patent and the university will get the rest.

The patent is licensed to a manufacturer. The product which this manufacturer makes does not work as well, by 75 %, as your prototype. You complain to the manufacturer but he ignores you. Instead he gets other university medical centers to repeat your original studies with the new equipment. As expected, it does not work as intended. Two published papers conclude that the technology is flawed and the equipment does not work.

What will you do?

© Springer Science+Business Media New York 2015
J.G. Brock-Utne, *Clinical Research*, DOI 10.1007/978-1-4939-2516-2_15

Answer/Solution

There is very little you can do unless you have a contract that says: "The final product must be to the inventor and/or patent holder's satisfaction."

Discussion

In this case the technology worked but the manufacturer's rendition of the device did not function as intended. The upshot was that the technology got discredited and the manufacturer went bankrupt.

Lesson

Never lose control of your invention and its development. This can/will end in disaster.

Chapter 16
Case 16: A Laboratory Lesson

You have collected blood samples from a clinical study. The patient's samples are taken to a laboratory and put in a freezer at −80 °C. When all samples are collected, they are to be analyzed. The study has been going on for 4 months.

One day when you are in the laboratory dropping off your samples, you notice painters at work in one part of the laboratory. You find out that they are going to paint the whole laboratory that week from Monday to Friday. The laboratory is very big with benches, shelves, a lot of electrical equipment, and of course several freezers.

Should you be concerned and if so what would you do?

© Springer Science+Business Media New York 2015
J.G. Brock-Utne, *Clinical Research*, DOI 10.1007/978-1-4939-2516-2_16

Answer/Solution

Make sure that the electrical cords to the freezers are not unplugged while they are painting.

Discussion

This happened to me. The painters unplugged the freezer with my samples on Friday afternoon for no apparent reason, and by Monday morning the samples were ruined.

What could have been done to prevent this from happening? Large notices on all sides of the freezers to state "Not to be unplugged" would hopefully have prevented it from happening. It is of paramount importance to inform everyone working in the laboratory that no electrical plug should be unplugged at any time.

Lesson

1. When people who do not work in the laboratory get access, they must be instructed as to what can and cannot be done.
2. Best of all is to check several times a day that everything is in order. If someone had checked the plugs on Friday afternoon, after the painters left, this would not have happened.

Chapter 17
Case 17: Before You Start Any Research

You just have been appointed to a university medical department with an expectation to do clinical research, but you have no grant to pay for your nonclinical time. The department gives you 1 day a week to do research. Not much, but this is a common arrangement until you show productivity with the time given. Should you be productive, the department may choose to further subsidize your research time.

After some thought you decide on a research area to pursue. What are the questions you should ask yourself before you embark on researching in your chosen area?

© Springer Science+Business Media New York 2015   35
J.G. Brock-Utne, *Clinical Research*, DOI 10.1007/978-1-4939-2516-2_17

Answer/Solution

A very good friend of mine, Dr. Alex Macario, who at the tender age of 42, became a full professor at Stanford University, answers the question most eloquently (http://www.medscape.com/viewarticle/727739). His many points are:

1. You do not want to pick an area where there are several other researchers that already have funding and/or 4 days a week to devote to the research topic you are considering. You will have a more difficult time getting recognized as an important contributor to this field. Also, the chances of getting funding will be limited since you are not a known entity.
2. Choosing an area that is understudied, such as children or parturient, but in your mind addresses important clinical questions, may make it difficult to get funding and/or time off from clinical duties to do research.
3. Having decided on a study, you must convince the head of the department to support you with either time or money or both. One way to do that is to get other colleagues to join in. The way to do that is to make an excellent joint presentation to both the head and to the department faculty. It is imperative to invite all of the department's faculty, so they understand what you are doing and why. This hopefully will generate some enthusiasm for the study and maybe get others to join in and help recruit patients. Remember: Involving others to help get the study done will also improve camaraderie. One of my many mentors, Jon Gjessing, Professor and Head of the Anesthesia Department at Rikshospitalet, Oslo, Norway, always said, "The more the merrier."
4. Don't just study one thing. As Alex says and I paraphrase him: "Don't put all your eggs in one basket—select 2 or 3 (preferably related) areas of investigation as an insurance should one fail."

    In Alex's case he decided to do research in operating room management. Having an MBA was a clear advantage. This was an area of research which no one studied when he started. However, the downside was that the federal government, industry, or other funding for this area was limited. As backup, he developed an interest in the economic assessment of new drugs and devices for use in surgical patients. This became his second line of investigation and was more likely to be funded as there was a budding interest in the field of cost-effectiveness analyses. Discussing these ideas above with a senior mentor can be helpful in part because the mentor may provide historical perspective on the research topic of interest.
5. Furthermore, I should add that you must have enough patients to complete the proposed trial in a reasonable time (see also Chap. 23).

Lesson

When picking your research subject, take your time and choose wisely.

Chapter 18
Case 18: An Offer of Employment: What to Look For

You have just finished your residency and have been active with clinical research. You have completed two abstracts and one paper is in press. You are excited about clinical research and decide to pursue an academic career. As luck would have it, three university departments want you to join them as a junior faculty. One of the departments that offer you a job is the one you trained in.

What are the many aspects you must consider prior to choosing?

© Springer Science+Business Media New York 2015   37
J.G. Brock-Utne, *Clinical Research*, DOI 10.1007/978-1-4939-2516-2_18

Answer/Solution

There are several aspects that you must consider prior to choosing your place of work:

1. It is a fact that each department, medical school, and hospital has individual strengths. It is important for you to identify what they are. Having done that you must ascertain how best these strengths can help you in your quest to become a leader in your chosen field of clinical research.
2. To accept a job in the place where you trained is a clear advantage for several reasons. You know the "setup," weaknesses and strengths, and the "culture" of the place. You have colleagues that you have worked with and it should be easy to find a mentor. Most importantly you will most likely get support from the head of the department.
3. If you accept a job in a new institution, it may prove difficult to get your research up and running. Nobody knows you and you may have difficulty finding a mentor. You may be competing with other researchers in your new department who are doing what you want to do. If that is the case and you feel that they do not want to cooperate with you, then don't take a job in that department. I have seen this happen with disastrous consequences for the "new boy." In that particular case, he was not given a renewal of a grant, which he got prior to coming to the new institution. But the main reason for his failure was that he did not get the help he was promised in the new place of employment.
4. In my experience it can take up to 2 years, after you commence work in a new department, before you are "up and running" with your research efforts.

Lesson

When choosing between job offers, take your time and check your facts.

Chapter 19
Case 19: What Should You Do?

As a junior faculty member, you are offered to participate in a simple clinical study. The study deals with the ability of anesthesiologists to estimate blood loss by just examining the blood on surgical sponges.

At the same time you are considering a large study for which you can apply for a grant. The study is something like the one in Case 6. You realize the study is broad and potentially difficult. But there is a lot of money and you believe that this larger study will catapult your career forward.

Since you will not have enough time to do them both, you must choose one or the other.

Which one should you do at this stage in your career?

© Springer Science+Business Media New York 2015
J.G. Brock-Utne, *Clinical Research*, DOI 10.1007/978-1-4939-2516-2_19

Answer/Solution

Choose the simple one.

Discussion

The reason is easy. It gives you an opportunity to get started quickly with a project and produce some results. It will also show everyone that you are keen to work hard and that you really like academic medicine. This simple study will exercise your skill as a researcher. You will have to write a protocol and consent form for the IRB and get the study approved by them. Being a simple study, this should be easy. The study should be finished in 2–3 weeks. When the study is finished, you can do the statistics, write the paper, and submit it to a journal. The latter is much more difficult than you think. If accepted, then you will have to deal with the revision. All in all, by doing small, quick studies, you will acquire knowledge in how clinical research is done and of course confirm that you find it interesting and fun.

I have seen so many juniors start studying large, complicated questions. They are too intricate and too time-consuming for a junior researcher. So often, I have seen them get frustrated, bored, and eventually give up.

If you are still in doubt as to which research project to choose, ask your mentor. I am sure he will agree that doing the small study, no matter how trivial it seems, should be done first.

Dr. Alex Macario and I did a small study [1]. This dealt with, as mentioned above, the estimation of a patient's blood loss by examining the surgical sponges. This little study, 10 years later received a National Institutes of Health (NIH) Small Business Innovation Research grant. The study looked at radio frequency identification tagging of surgical sponges. It is important to realize that every year, hundreds of surgical sponges are left behind in patients after surgery.

Lesson

Small studies should be done first before embarking on more extensive studies. The fact that you can rapidly see the fruits of your labor when your work is accepted for publication will prove a great satisfaction to you and spur you on to further clinical research.

Reference

1. Macario A, Brock-Utne JG. Anesthesiologist overestimate blood loss in both dry and wet surgical sponges. Can J Anaesth. 1994;41:1017–8.

Chapter 20
Case 20: Who to Trust

You are an assistant professor in a large university department. As a keen, budding researcher you have attended all the department's research meetings and have partaken in the discussions. An interesting clinical research project is presented by a senior researcher in the department. You show an obvious interest. The study involves measuring vital signs during general anesthesia and taking blood samples for bioactive agents. The next day the senior researcher stops you in the hall and asks you if you would like to be involved in the study. You are delighted. Your main job will be to measure the bioactive agents after all the samples have been collected. He has a laboratory technician who will teach you how to do the various laboratory tests. The senior researcher tells you that he has everything you need; he just wants you to do the work. He promises you first authorship. You thank him and tell him that you will go to the laboratory to ascertain how difficult it will be to learn the various assays, since you have no laboratory training. After spending 2–3 h with the technician, you realize that learning the techniques will take time and effort, but you are confident you can do it. You are however concerned that the technician may not have time to help you, should you need assistance from time to time. Also you have no understanding of the possible clinical importance of this study.

You consult another assistant professor in the department. He has been there 1 year longer than you. He has not done much research and is at present not engaged in any. You conclude that he does not seem to have the interest, but you ask him anyway. He tells you that he would not do it based on what you tell him. He also tells you that he has heard that the senior researcher can be difficult to work with at times. The latter is news to you and you can hardly believe it.

Based on the above, you call on the senior researcher and tell him that you do not accept his kind offer.

But is this the right answer?

© Springer Science+Business Media New York 2015   41
J.G. Brock-Utne, *Clinical Research*, DOI 10.1007/978-1-4939-2516-2_20

Answer/Solution

This is not the right answer.

Discussion

This happened to be a great friend of mine. He went and told the senior researcher that unfortunately he could not do the study. Unbeknown to my friend, the assistant professor, whom he had consulted, went and offered to help with the study. The senior researcher said he would be happy to have him participate. Several months later my friend found out what had happened and asked the assistant professor why he decided to work on this project. The answer was that he had thought about it and decided it was a good idea. The assistant professor completed the study, albeit with much delay on his part, but he did get a publication out of it.

Lesson

1. Do not turn down a research offer from a senior member of staff. You must realize that the senior member has identified you as a person that has the potential to do research. To join his team is invaluable; as if you are successful, he will serve as a mentor to you.
2. Be careful when taking advice from a colleague of the same standing as you. It is better to ask advice from senior members of staff in the department, who are unlikely to be in competition with you.
3. If you don't know anything about the study and its objective, find out.
4. Never be worried about learning new skills. My grandfather always said, "They can take everything away from you, except what you have learned."
5. In the above case, the publication was published in a leading journal. It was considered so important that the editor of the journal had an expert write a glowing editorial related to the study.
6. Finally, *The New York Times* ran an article on it and the researchers were invited to be interviewed on Good Morning America.

Chapter 21
Case 21: Elementary

You are doing a clinical research study to establish if using your personal ultraviolet (UV) camera can make the intravenous (IV) insertion of an IV catheter easier than using the department's ultrasound. The study is done in the preoperative holding area, in a separate room. The study is nearly completed and no clear advantage of the UV camera can be ascertained.

One day, having completed a study on a patient, you leave, as is your practice, both the ultrasound machine and the UV camera in the study area and take the patient to the operating room.

Is there anything wrong with this picture?

© Springer Science+Business Media New York 2015   43
J.G. Brock-Utne, *Clinical Research*, DOI 10.1007/978-1-4939-2516-2_21

Answer/Solution

Never leave any equipment unattended, even if it's an equipment that you think would be of no interest to anyone.

Discussion

The above case happened to us. A good friend and researcher Dr. Michael Chen and I had the UV camera stolen from the preoperative area. Nobody had seen anything and the camera was never found. The study came to an abrupt halt. Fortunately, as mentioned, the UV camera was shown to have no clear advantage over ultrasound. The loss of the camera was not devastating

Far worse was when I lost a personal computer in a procedure room, with data from an 8-month study. This was in 2000 and I did not have the knowledge or thought to back up my data. It was shocking that this should happen in a work environment where you think you can trust everyone. Now I look after my research equipment like a hawk and I back up everything.

Lesson

If your research equipment cannot be continuously monitored, then it must be supervised by someone you trust. If it is not being utilized, it must be locked away.

Chapter 22
Case 22: Never Give Up

You have submitted a paper to a large North American medical journal. It is the opinion of you and your coworkers that it is a great paper. Over 100 patients were included, and the paper shows interesting and previously unpublished results.

But the paper is not accepted. The criticisms are vague; the tone of the review is disrespectful and the language damning. In short you are told that the results would be of very little interest to the practicing clinician. You do not agree but feel the editor and the reviewers must be correct.

Based on the above, you do not attempt to resubmit to another journal.

Less than 2 years later, a paper dealing with the same question is published in the same journal. Of note is the fact that whole paragraphs are identical to your submission which had been rejected.

What did you do wrong?

© Springer Science+Business Media New York 2015
J.G. Brock-Utne, *Clinical Research*, DOI 10.1007/978-1-4939-2516-2_22

Answer/Solution

You should have resubmitted to another journal. Never give up, especially if you think it is a worthwhile paper.

Discussion

This happened to us around 1984. The most likely reason for the rejection of our paper was that one or maybe two of the reviewers were working on the same question. After rejecting our paper, they published their findings on the same topic.

So what did we do about this plagiarism? We did nothing. We believed that writing to the editor could jeopardize any future submission from us and an accusation of plagiarism was a serious allegation.

In 2014 I submitted a letter to the editor dealing with the above experience. My letter was entitled: "Another example of plagiarism. Hopefully rare." The letter was in response to recent articles on plagiarizing in their journal. The editor and reviewers did not want to publish it, as they claimed that this would never happen today.

The reasons given were the following:

1. Editors and reviewers are now held liable. As a reviewer you agree to and sign a contract stating that you will treat all manuscripts in review as confidential documents and not disclose its contents outside the context of the review process.
2. A written confidentiality agreement between the reviewer and the journal includes the following statement: "that I agree that I shall not disclose, divulge, transfer or otherwise convey to the journal confidential information, directly or indirectly, to any person or entity other than to individuals who have signed confidentiality agreements. I further acknowledge that all information related to editorial performance is confidential information." This means a reviewer should not use information or wordings in your submitted manuscript in any of his/her work.

Had our paper been published, before the publication that plagiarized us then, proving plagiarism would have been easy.

One can only hope that all journals, including online journals, adhere to the trust you have in them when you submit your work. It is obvious that reviewers or editors who commit such plagiarism should be dismissed. But if it is the editor in chief who is the culprit, then how is he/she fired?

I have to say that most of my contact with reviewers and editors (over 46 years now) has been respectful and civil. Maybe one lesson here is that if you get an unprofessional reply, take the good points that are made for not accepting your work and incorporate those into your resubmission to another journal.

Lesson

Don't give up if your paper gets rejected. Resubmit to another journal. This is especially true if you think the results will advance the science of medicine and possibly improve patient care.

Chapter 23
Case 23: How Long Should a Study Go On?

You have just been recruited as a young assistant professor in a clinical department. An associate professor in the same department seeks you out as he is keen for you to participate in an ongoing industry-sponsored research project. The study has been ongoing for 12 months, but only 40 % of the required numbers of patients have been enrolled.

You review the protocol, the consent form, and the data sheet and do a literature search and decide that the study has merit. You interview the two nursing coordinators who are involved with the study. They seem a bit frustrated. Added to this, it doesn't seem that there are enough patients admitted to the hospital with the disease process you are investigating. The associate professor tells you not to worry as the hospital is in the process of hiring another specialist who is very well known in the field. This he tells you will increase the patient population for the study. He also offers you first authorship, should you be successful.

What would you do? Accept or decline?

© Springer Science+Business Media New York 2015
J.G. Brock-Utne, *Clinical Research*, DOI 10.1007/978-1-4939-2516-2_23

Answer/Solution

Decline, unless you can:

1. Verify that the specialist is coming to work there soon
2. Hire two new nursing coordinators

Discussion

The above happened to a friend of mine. He accepted the offer, but the study was never completed. This was mainly because there was a lack of suitable patients since the new specialist never came. Since the study dragged on, the nurses involved with the study got bored, lost focus, and worst of all they started to "cut corners" by enrolling patients that, by the study criteria, should not have been included.

Had my friend had enough patients and new and enthusiastic research nurses, he could have finished the study.

Lesson

There will be pitfalls when you take over a research project that is not completed within the stipulated time. The main reasons often are that the people who have been involved with the study get bored and lose focus. I suggest that in such a case as the one above, it would be essential to employ new and enthusiastic nurses to help you complete the study.

In my experience, a clinical study lasting more than 12 months will rarely be completed.

Chapter 24
Case 24: What to Do?

As a clinical instructor in anesthesiology, you have an ongoing study in the Interventional Radiology (IR) Suite. Patients in the IR Suite routinely get cold during general anesthesia. This is because the patient is usually fully exposed and the rooms are cold. Since X-rays are being used, water blankets can't be employed. Air convection surface heaters (Bair Hugger) are of little use because they cover up the body and will be in the way of the IR physician.

In an effort to prevent hypothermia to the patient, you have obtained an IRB approval to study a new noninvasive surface heater applied to the limbs. The study was started 6 months ago and involves measuring the patient's tympanic temperature at the start of the anesthetic and in the recovery room. All patients are to get the heating device, and these results will initially be compared to historical data. In this way, one will quickly see if the device makes the patients warmer in the recovery room.

But unfortunately, you and your colleague from the department of anesthesiology are losing interest as it is proving difficult to get the patients to consent to the study.

You fail to understand why there should be such a problem getting consent from the patients for such a simple and noninvasive project. You suggest paying the patients, but there is no money. If there had been, it would have necessitated a major change to the IRB consent form, and the research would have been delayed by at least 2 months. You ask an associate professor in the Department of Anesthesiology for suggestions on how to increase your informed consent success rate.

What do you think the associate professor will suggest?

© Springer Science+Business Media New York 2015
J.G. Brock-Utne, *Clinical Research*, DOI 10.1007/978-1-4939-2516-2_24

Answer/Solution

He suggests that you involve one or more of the IR physicians to be authors in the study. They know the patients and the patients have bonded with them. In this case that is all that was needed to get the project completed in a timely manner.

Discussion

Always invite anyone who can be helpful in your research endeavor to join a project as an author. By involving enthusiastic members from other departments in your research, you increase your chances of success. The people you involve must be enthusiastic because if they are not, the study will probably not be completed. In the above case, you should explain the purpose of the study to the IR doctors. Don't send an e-mail, etc. You must go and see them. Remind them of the dangers of hypothermia and tell them that the study is hoping to prove that this noninvasive heating device may help in preventing hypothermia.

I have found that this type of research cooperation can often improve morale and promote team spirit between the various specialties.

Lesson

If you are relying on other health care providers, perhaps from a different department, to help you in your study, make sure you invite them to be authors.

Chapter 25
Case 25: To What Journal Should You Send Your Work?

Many years ago we published a study entitled: "Does maternal medication temporarily affect neonatal neurobehavior?" The study started in partnership with a prominent German neonatal psychologist Brigitte Niestroj from Berlin who was spending a year working with us in Durban. At the time, I was working in King Edward VIII Hospital, Durban, where we were doing between 32,000 and 36,000 deliveries which included 6–8,000 Cesarean sections a year. Brigitte was interested in the possible effect of maternal medication on the neonate's neurobehavior function. Together we modified the Brazelton neurobehavioral scale and made it much simpler, less time-consuming, and less exhausting for the newborn [1].

We studied healthy newborns at 2–4 h and at 24 h after birth. Many of the mothers came to deliver their babies in the hospital so late before delivery that there was no time to give any medication before the baby was delivered, while another group would get medication for labor pain. Hence we had two groups. Brigitte was blinded as to the presence or absence of maternal medication. The results showed that tone, reflexes, and rooting score all decreased at 2–4 h with medication (17.2 vs.19.2) $p <0.005$, but no difference was detected at 24 h. We recommended that this scale be used as a research tool in obstetric anesthesia.

We were delighted with the results, but to which journal or journals do you suggest we should submit our paper for publication?

© Springer Science+Business Media New York 2015
J.G. Brock-Utne, *Clinical Research*, DOI 10.1007/978-1-4939-2516-2_25

Answer/Solution

Submit the paper to a neonatal, neurobehavioral, or obstetric journal.

Discussion

In general, where to publish your work is dependent on the research that you are doing and what the results and conclusions are. It is important to review many journals to establish where previous work, like yours, has been published. In this case it would have been correct to attempt to send it to the journal where Brazelton first published his work. Most likely Brazelton himself would be one of the reviewers. If he liked it, good. If he did not, he would probably give very good feedback. Be aware that you must, in this case, quote Dr. Brazelton correctly!

In our case, we published the work in the South African Medical Journal (SAMJ) [2]. We chose that journal because Brigitte wanted a quick publication for her CV as she was going back to Germany. Submitting it to SAMJ was a big mistake. It was the wrong journal to choose as few people of consequence in this field read it.

We realized too late that we should have sent our work to a more specialized journal where the readership would have been more appreciative of our manuscript. We made a real blunder by publishing in a more general medical journal. Although our "scale" was shown in our study to offer a simple practical approach in assessing the presence or absence of maternal medication on a neonate, it was never universally adapted. By publishing it in a general medical journal we put our work in a coffin.

It is interesting that 2 months after our publication, another neonatal scoring system (NACS) similar to ours was published [3]. An editorial by Tronick [4] found "potential pitfalls and predicted that sensitivity (and perhaps validity) will be found wanting." NACS is used to this day while ours is not. Congratulations goes to the editor of Anesthesiology at the time [5] who recognized that the work was most likely in its developmental stage and that publication like this "should not await maturation." In 2000, Brockhurst et al. [6] conclude that "Research is needed to establish the reliability and validity of the NACS." The editorial by Camann and Brazelton [7] states: "For now, the NACS will certainly continue to appear like barnacles on a ships masthead in many studies of obstetric anesthetic. If NACS does nothing else, at least it forces us to remember that neonatal concerns are an important part of obstetric anesthesia. That in itself is a worthwhile goal."

But a real blunder, with historical and political consequence was Gregor Mendel who published "Laws on Heredity" in 1865 [8]. The journal he selected can only, even at that time, be described as an obscure journal. Very few people read it. The work lay dormant until early 1900, more than 35 years after it was first published. The lack of known heredity science led both Stalin and Hitler to advocate political justification in killing certain people [9]. It is imperative that all researchers should keep their readers/editors in mind when preparing a manuscript for a specific journal.

Be wary of new journals as they often have a lower standard than established ones. This is because new journals may have to accept most articles that are submitted to them in order to fill their pages. Also be aware that these journals may not survive. If that happens your work could be very difficult to access in the future by other researchers.

When reviewing your prospective journal, try and get an idea of its reputation for giving a thorough and fair editorial review with helpful refereeing. The "turn-around" time from submission to when you hear back from the journal is also important. (I have personally waited over 10 months for a reply and hence never sent more work to that journal). Some researchers look at the editorial board to ascertain if the editorial system is fair and unbiased. The editor in chief bears the responsibility for the journal's contents. His or her reputation will suffer should the standard be deemed mediocre. Also remember to read and follow the instructions to the authors. This may help you decide if this journal is the right one for your work. Information as to length and layout of the articles and the various journal policies will save you a lot of time later, should the paper be accepted. Many editors get upset if you have not followed their detailed instructions and this can play a major part in them not accepting your paper.

According to Lanier [10] most authors pay little attention to where to submit their work. Too much reliance is made on mentors, colleagues, friends, or on the past relationships they have had with a journal. Lanier says that when the author is looking for a journal, he/she should ask and I quote:

1. Do I have a high-quality message?
2. Who will benefit from hearing the message?
3. Is the journal I have chosen the right "conduit" to reach my intended audience?

I recommend you to read this presentation: Dr. W. L. Lanier about the Editorial Process for Peer-Reviewed Medical Literature: The Journal's Point of View [10].

Lesson

Be very careful where you send your work. If you have your manuscript accepted in the wrong journal, this will often mean that it will not be read by the people you want to inform. In addition, it will not have the desired impact in clinical practice.

References

1. Brazelton TB. Neonatal behavioral assessment scale London/Philadelphia/Heinemann/ Lippincott. 1973
2. Brock-Utne JG. Does maternal medication temporarily affect neonatal neurobehavior? South Afr Med J. 1982;62:985–9.

3. Amiel-Tison C, Barrier G, Snider SM, Levinson G, Hughes SC, Stefani SJ. A new neurologic and adaptive capacity scoring system for evaluating obstetric medication in full term newborns. Anesthesiology. 1982;56:340–50.

4. Tronick E. A critique of the neonatal neurologic and adaptive capacity score (NACS). Anesthesiology. 1982;56:338–9.

5. Michenfelder JD. Accept, revise, reject or punt: an example of the latter. Anesthesiology. 1982;56:337.

6. Brockhurst NJ, Littleford JA, Halpern SH. The neurologic and adaptive capacity score. Anesthesiology. 2000;92:237–46.

7. Camann W, Brazelton TB. Use and abuse of neonatal neurobehavioral testing. Anesthesiology. 2000;92:3–5.

8. Mendel JG. *Versuche über Pflanzenhybriden* Verhandlungen des naturforschenden Vereines in Brünn, Bd. IV für das Jahr, 1865. Abhandlungen. 1866; 3–47. For the English translation, see: Druery CT, Bateson W. Experiments in plant hybridization. J R Horticult Soc. 1901; 26:1–32. Retrieved 9 Oct 2009.

9. Cornwell J. Hitler's scientists: science, war, and the devil's pact. London: Penguin Group; 2003.

10. Lanier WL. The editorial process for peer-reviewed medical literature: the journal's point of view. A Review lecture given at International, Anesthesia, Research, (IARS Society). 2006

Chapter 26
Case 26: A Drug-Sponsored Trial

You have completed a drug-sponsored trial. The agreement was for the pharmaceutical company to pay the department several thousand dollars in installments for the work done. The money was used for a research nurse and to pay the laboratory for analyzing blood samples. At the conclusion of the study, the results were to be submitted to the sponsor. At that point, the last installment was to be paid.

In this case, the results were not to the company's liking. They didn't want to have them published and were so unhappy with them that they withheld the last payment.

Left with this situation what would you do now?

© Springer Science+Business Media New York 2015   57
J.G. Brock-Utne, *Clinical Research*, DOI 10.1007/978-1-4939-2516-2_26

Answer/Solution

Read the contract again.

Discussion

There are two responses, depending if you have:

1. Agreed that the sponsor will decide if the manuscript is to be published or not.
     If you agreed to that, then there is nothing to be done. This happened to me. The university agreed with the sponsor and therefore prevented me from submitting it. The last installment was not paid and the paper did not get published. Luckily I had some extra research money to cover the last study expenses.
2. NOT agreed with the above clause, but the sponsor still tells you not to publish and also withholds the last installment; then there are several things you must do.

   A. If the study is of clinical relevance, you must publish. If you had shown the drug to be next to useless and previous studies shown to be very effective, then it is imperative to seek publication.
   B. As regards to nonpayment, then you must:

      (1) Tell the head of the department
      (2) Tell the IRB
      (3) Tell the Dean's office
      (4) Tell the University Ombudsman

This latter approach should provoke such a reaction that the company will pay up.

Lesson

1. Always read the contract in detail, especially as it relates to payment conditions.
2. Never agree that you will abide by a company's decision to publish or not. If the results are important to patient care, then you must publish. If you don't, patient care could be compromised and you would have wasted valuable research time.

Chapter 27
Case 27: The Difference Between Research and Quality Assurance/Improvement

Federal Regulations [1] define research as "a systematic investigation, including research development, testing and evaluation, designed to develop or contribute to generalizable knowledge," while medical quality assurance/improvement (QI) projects are defined as "reviewing patient care, identification of clinical problems and the evaluation of actions directed to correct or prevent them from occurring."

Here is an example of a QI manuscript that was submitted for publication as a research project to a leading anesthesia journal. The object of the QI was to examine the safety of concurrent use of epidural and intravenous opiates in pediatric cancer patients. The retrospective reviews of the charts were approved by the institution's IRB as a quality improvement (QI) project.

The charts were reviewed every 4 h to establish the child's pain, level of consciousness, vital signs, motor function, and pulse oximetry. No CO_2 capnography was done. The end point was respiratory depression. This was defined as the need for naloxone or endotracheal intubation and ventilation. Intravenous opiates were given prn.

The study concluded that the supplementation of epidural opiates with IV opiates was safe in this population group. You are asked by the editor of the journal to review this paper.

Based on the information given above, will you accept or reject this paper?

© Springer Science+Business Media New York 2015
J.G. Brock-Utne, *Clinical Research*, DOI 10.1007/978-1-4939-2516-2_27

Answer/Solution

Reject.

Discussion

The main reason for my rejection was that the observations were done retrospectively every 4 h, which did not connect with the timing of IV opiates. Patients can stop breathing when IV opiates are given to them while receiving concurrent epidural opiates. Hence this paper poses an important question: is the concurrent use of epidural and intravenous opiates in pediatric cancer patients safe? This question is not answered by this type of study. Other researchers agree [2]. Only, a prospective study with informed consent by the parents can potentially answer this question.

In this case the researchers had wanted to do a prospective trial and asked the IRB for a waiver of informed consent. This is because they thought rightly that it would have been a challenge to obtain informed consent from the parents for studying potential respiratory distress in their child.

The Federal Regulations (detailed in 45CFR46.116(d) [3] state that a waiver of informed consent can be made when *all* of the following conditions are present:

a. The research involves no more than minimal risk to the subjects.
b. The waiver or alteration will not adversely affect the rights and welfare of the subjects.
c. The research could not practicably be carried out without this waiver or alteration.
d. Whenever appropriate, subject will be provided with additional pertinent information after participation.

It is therefore obvious that a prospective study with a waiver of informed consent for this study would not be approved by any institutional review board. These questions will therefore probably never be answered satisfactorily.

I recommend the readers to follow the dialogue between Murphy GS et al. who published a QI study in anesthesia and analgesia in 2009 [4] and Anderson JR and Schonfeld T [5] who felt that their study was a research study and not a QI. The reply from Murphy GS et al. [6] and from Steve Shafer (the Editor of A&A) is worth reading as Dr. Shafer recognizes the difficulty sometimes in distinguishing between QI or QA (quality assurance) and research [7].

Furthermore, a similar prospective study by Overdyk et al. [8] recommends that continuous respiratory monitoring should be considered for the safe administration of PCA. This is because respiratory depression can progress to respiratory arrest if undetected.

Lesson

If you consider publishing QI results, then you need to ascertain if a waiver of informed consent can be obtained and your IRB has no objection to you attempting to publish this study.

References

1. U.S. Government Printing office; Code of Federal Regulations. Title 45 public welfare, vol 1, Dept of Health & Human Services, Definitions 46.102; 2002. p. 107. http://edocket.access.gpo.gov/cfr_2002/octqtr/pdf/45crr46.102.pdf.
2. Overdyk F, Carter R, Maddox R. New JCAHO pain standard bigger threat to patient safety than envisioned. Anesth Analg. 2006;102:1596–7.
3. U.S. Government Printing office; Code of Federal Regulations. Title 45 public welfare, vol 1, Dept of Health & Human Services, General Requirements for Informed Consent, 46.116; 2003. p. 117. http://edocket.access.gpo.gov/cfr_2003/octqtr/pdf/45cfr46.116.pdf.
4. Murphy GS, Szokol JW, Marymont JH, Greenberg SB, Avram KJ, Vender JS. Residual neuromuscular blockade and critical respiratory events in the postanesthesia care unit. Anesth Analg. 2008;107:130–7.
5. Anderson JG, Schonfeld T. Research, not quality assurance. Anesth Analg. 2009;108:376.
6. Murphy GS, Scokol JW, Marymont JE, Greenberg SB, Avram MJ, Vender JS. Research, not quality assurance. Anesth Analg. 2009;108:376–7.
7. Shafer SL. Research, not quality assurance. Anesth Analg. 2009;108:377–8.
8. Overdyk FJ, Carter R, Maddox RR, Callura J, Herrin AE, Henriquez C. Continuous oximetry/capnometry monitoring reveals frequent desaturation and bradypnea during patient controlled analgesia. Anesth Analg. 2007;105:412–8.

Chapter 28
Case 28: Stopping a Clinical Study

We started a prospective study entitled:

"A comparison of open versus laparoscopic gastric bypass operations in morbidly obese patients".

The same surgeon was doing both open and laparoscopic surgeries and the anesthetic technique was the same. After 20 patients, it became apparent that the patients who had the laparoscopic bypass procedure did much better postoperatively. This group had a shorter time to discharge from the recovery room, to take clear liquids, and a shorter hospital stay. There was also improved patient satisfaction and of course reduced hospital cost.

What would you do in this circumstance? Stop the trial or carry on?

© Springer Science+Business Media New York 2015
J.G. Brock-Utne, *Clinical Research*, DOI 10.1007/978-1-4939-2516-2_28

Answer/Solution

We stopped the trial early, mainly at the behest of the surgeon who felt strongly that he did not feel it was ethical to carry on.

We therefore took an additional historical data randomly from seven patients, who had undergone open gastric bypass operations. This made a total of 13 patients in group 1. We then compared these results to those obtained from the 14 prospectively laparoscopic gastric bypass surgeries. The results were amazing. All the above parameters reached statistical significance $p < 0.05$ to $p < 0.001$ using a two-tailed t-test of two samples [1]. Not only was there a statistical significance, but the results were clinically relevant as, for example, the hospital stay was reduced from 6.8 days (group 1 open) to 4.5 days (group 2 laparoscopic)

Discussion

This study started as a clinical study with IRB approval with the same surgeon doing both operations in a prospective randomized trial. However, after 20 patients had been enrolled, the surgeon Dr. Mark Vierra felt that it was not ethical to carry on as the patients who had the laparoscopic procedure were doing much better post-operatively compared to those who underwent the open procedure.

Several researchers have indicated that there are times when a clinical trial must be stopped before all subjects have entered the trial [2–4]. This should occur when it is obvious to the researchers that there is a clear benefit with one treatment modality over another or harm is being inflicted on the patients. But Myles [2] suggest that reviewing data from a study that one is considering stopping can lead to the wrong conclusions of effect, since a type I error can occur. He suggests that an independent data and safety monitoring committee (DSMC) should be called in to review the study. The object of the DSMC is to make sure that the interests of patients enrolled in the study and of those that might be included are protected. Stopping a trial early should not be taken lightly as DSMC must consider if the trial findings to date may change or not change clinical practice. In our case [1] we felt that our report did change clinical practice for the better. Personally I think the decision to stop a clinical trial early is common sense when it is obvious that one technique is better than the other. I am skeptical as the suggestion to establish a DSMC in hospitals that do research. Where would you get qualified members to sit on such a committee unless the DSMC is in a large medical center? Just consider, who the members of this committee should be? They must have done years of clinical research, being experts in statistical methods, knowledge of epidemiology, and have an ethical understanding of clinical research.

However, there are several examples when clinical trials have been stopped early and where subsequent research has come to different conclusions from those that stopped the trials [5–7]. In some instances, the new research has either refuted the conclusion or questioned whether the treatment was effective or even harmful.

There are other reasons for stopping a trial. For instance, people get tired, lose interest (see Chap. 10), no more funds, there are no suitable patients, and/or new evidence suggests that the research treatment may cause harm.

Lesson

In our case we started with a prospective randomized trial but ended up with a mixture, as we had to use historical data. We got only an abstract out of our work but feel that it was the correct decision, as our results had an impact on patient care.

References

1. Brock-Utne JG, Ohayon E, Lemmens HJM, Brodsky JB, Vierra M. Open versus laparoscopic gastric bypass surgery. Analysis of select recovery parameters. Anesth Analg. 2001;92:S158.
2. Myles PS. Stopping trials early. Br J Anaesth. 2013;111:133–5.
3. Korn EL, Freidlin B, Mooney M. Stopping or reporting early for positive results in randomized clinical trials: the National Cancer Institute Cooperative Group experience from 1990 to 2005. J Clin Oncol. 2009;27:1712–21.
4. Pocock SJ. When to stop a clinical trial. Br Med J. 1992;305:235–40.
5. Yeager M, Glass D, Neff R, Brinck-Johnsen T. Epidural anesthesia and analgesia in high risk surgical patients. Anesthesiology. 1987;66:729–36.
6. Mashour GA, Shanks A, Tremper KK, et al. Prevention of intraoperative awareness with explicit recall in an unselected surgical population: randomized comparative effectiveness trial. Anesthesiology. 2012;117:717–25.
7. Poldermans D, Boersma E, Bax J. The effect of bisoprolol on perioperative mortality and myocardial infarction in high risk patients undergoing vascular surgery. N Engl J Med. 1999;341:1788–94.

Chapter 29
Case 29: Controversy

Many years ago a professor of gastroenterology, Dr. Mike Moshal, told us that the intravenous injection of atropine will decrease the lower esophageal sphincter (LES) tone [1]. In all our anesthesia textbooks, at that time, atropine was reported to increase the LES tone [2]. After the lecture, I told him so. He said: "Well that is interesting. Please give me the reference."

A few days later I went to his lab and gave him the reference. After reading the reference, he said that he did not believe that atropine increased LES but rather decreased it as he knew and respected these researchers [1].

So is that the end of the story or what will you do?

© Springer Science+Business Media New York 2015
J.G. Brock-Utne, *Clinical Research*, DOI 10.1007/978-1-4939-2516-2_29

Answer/Solution

Repeat the study if possible and remember that controversial results are great research opportunities.

Discussion

Professor Moshal had the latest esophageal measuring devices, and he and his staff, especially Dr. G.E. Dimopoulos, had been trained in the accepted methods of interpretation of the pressure changes in the stomach, LES, and esophagus. I therefore suggested to him that this was a worthwhile research project especially since the anesthesia studies were done in cadavers [2]. That convinced him. We created a team of gastroenterologists, obstetricians, anesthesiologists, and technicians, and we successfully concluded many studies in relation to the acid aspiration and the effects of many anesthesia drugs on the lower esophageal sphincter [3–19].

Lesson

Controversial studies can be a "gold mine" of research opportunities.

References

1. Lind JF, Crispin JS, McIver DK. The effect of atropine on the gastroesophageal sphincter. Can J Physiol Pharm. 1968;48:233–8.
2. Clark CG, Riddoch ME. Observation on the human cardia at operation. Br J Anaesth. 1962;34:875–83.
3. Brock-Utne JG, Rubin J, Downing JW, Dimopoulos GE, Moshal MG, Naicker M. The administration of metoclopramide with atropine. (A drug interaction effect on the gastro-oesphageal sphincter in man). Anaesthesia. 1976;31:1186–90.
4. Brock-Utne JG, Rubin J, McAravey R, Dow TGB, Welman S, Dimopoulos GE, et al. The effect of hyoscine and atropine on the lower oesphaegal sphincter. Anaesth Intens Care. 1977;3:223–5.
5. Brock-Utne JG, Rubin J, Welman S, Dimopoulos GE, Moshal MG, Downing JW. The effect of glycopyrrolate (Robinul) on the lower oesophageal sphincter. Can Anaesth Soc J. 1978;25:144–6.
6. Dow TGB, Brock-Utne JG, Rubin J, Welman S, Dimopoulos GE, Moshal MG. The effect of atropine on the lower esophageal sphincter in late pregnancy. Obstet Gynecol. 1978;51:426–30.
7. Brock-Utne JG, Dow TGB, Welman S, Dimopoulos GE, Moshal MG. The effect of metoclopramide on the lower oesophageal sphincter in late pregnancy. Anaesth Intens Care. 1978;6:26–8.
8. Brock-Utne JG, Rubin J, Welman S, Dimopoulos GE, Moshal MG, Downing JW. The action of commonly used antiemetics on the lower oesophageal sphincter. Br J Anaesth. 1978;50:295–7.

9. Brock-Utne JG, Downing JW, Welman S, Dimopoulos GE, Moshal MG. Lower esophageal sphincter tone during reversal of neuromuscular blockade by atropine and neostigmine. Anesth Analg. 1978;57:171–4.
10. Brock-Utne JG. Reversal of neuromuscular blockade by glycopyrrolate and neostigmine. Anaesthesia. 1978;34:620–2.
11. Brock-Utne JG, Downing JW, Dimopoulos GE, Rubin J, Moshal MG. Effect of domperidone on lower esophageal sphincter tone in late pregnancy. Anesthesiology. 1980;52:321–3.
12. Brock-Utne JG. Domperidone antagonizes the relaxant effect of atropine on the lower esophageal sphincter. Anesth Analg. 1980;59:921–4.
13. Brock-Utne JG, Dow TGB, Dimopoulos GE, Welman S, Downing JW, Moshal MG. Gastric and lower oesophageal sphincter (LOS) pressures in early pregnancy. Br J Anaesth. 1981;53:381–4.
14. Brock-Utne JG, Dimopoulos GE, Downing JW, Moshal MG. Gastro-Conray does not alter resting lower oesphageal sphincter pressure in normal human subjects. S Afr Med J. 1982;61:22–3.
15. Brock-Utne JG, Dowing JW, Dimopoulos GE, Moshal MG. Effect of metoclopramide given before atropine sulphate on lower oesophageal sphincter (LOS) tone. S Afr Med J. 1982;61:564–7.
16. Rubin J, Brock-Utne JG, Dimopoulos GE, Downing JW, Moshal MG. Flunitrazepam IV increases and diazepam IV decreases the lower oesophageal sphincter tone. Anaesth Intens Care. 1982;10:130–2.
17. Brock-Utne JG, Downing JW. The effect of 50% nitrous oxide in oxygen on lower oesophageal sphincter tone. Anaesthesia. 1983;38:383–5.
18. Rubin J, Brock-Utne JG, Downing JW. Intravenous midazolam does not change lower oesophageal sphincter tone. S Afr Med J. 1983;64:1024–5.
19. Brock-Utne JG, Downing JW, Humphrey D. Effect of ranitidine given before atropine sulphate on lower oesophageal sphincter tone. Anesth Intens Care. 1984;12:140–2.

Chapter 30
Case 30: The *P* Value

If the statistical analysis of your research work shows a *p*-value of $p < 0.05$, then this is an indication that your results are statistically significant. Furthermore, the paper produced has a great chance of getting accepted for publication. Also, if this was a pilot study, then you may be eligible for funding.

A young colleague proposes a clinical study to determine the onset time of tourniquet pain following a Bier block. Animal studies have shown that the addition of glucose 5 % to a local anesthetic solution (lidocaine 0.5 %) decreases corneal animal pain [1]. He has worked out that he needs to study 80 patients to get a *p*-value of <0.05.

He concludes the study and the desired *p*-value is achieved. In the result section, he only states that the patients with glucose in the Bier block solution reported tourniquet pain 7 min later than the pure lidocaine group. The study was accepted for publication in an open journal with some revision. At this point your colleague shows you the paper. After having read it, you ask him if he believes that the results are clinically meaningful even though they are statistically significant.

What do you think?

© Springer Science+Business Media New York 2015
J.G. Brock-Utne, *Clinical Research*, DOI 10.1007/978-1-4939-2516-2_30

Answer/Solution

When writing a paper do not only comment on the statistically significant change found but also make a statement as to if these results are clinically meaningful.

Discussion

We did a small similar clinical Bier block study and found what is described above. An abstract was produced [2]. We then decided to increase the sample size in the hope to show more of a significant clinical change. Unfortunately, with a larger study we did not find a significant difference, and the difference in the onset of pain was only 4 min: not clinically significant.

It is a fact that researchers often imply that a statistically significant result also means that it is clinically important. Even if you have a large sample and get a significant *p*-value that does not mean that the finding will improve patient care.

Dr. Zeev Kain [3] has outlined what he believes is important for a researcher to answer when investigating new treatments:

1. Could the findings of the clinical trial be solely a result of a chance occurrence (i.e., is it statistical significance)?
2. How rare is the difference between the primary end points of the study groups (i.e., impact of treatment, effect of size)?
3. Is the difference of primary end points between groups meaningful to a patient (i.e., clinical significance)?

In his article, Kain [3] mentions the use of confidence intervals (CI). This has been suggested by some [4]. But as Feinstein [5] says, getting a $p < 0.05$ is the same as a 95 % CI. It is worth noting that it can be used to estimate the size of differences between groups [6]. CI is not widely used today, and the use of the boundary of accepting or rejecting the null hypothesis is more common. The latter was introduced by Fisher [7, 8]. He arbitrarily set the boundary at $P = 0.05$. It is important to realize that the *p*-value does not take into account the size and clinical significance of the clinical effect seen. Hence, a large sample size study giving a small effect can have the same *p*-value as a large effect in a small sample size study. Further reading on this topic is suggested [9–17].

A most amusing and educational study is produced by Greenberg et al. [16]. In it he shows the unexpected association between rain and the annual meeting of the Society for Pediatric Anesthesia. He found a statistically significant *p*-value of 0.006. According to Drs. Shafer and Dexter [17], he satisfied all the requirements of correct statistical analysis. It is as Drs. Shafer and Dexter state: "…complete nonsense. It shows an example of publication bias, retrospective bias, and the questionable reproducibility of even highly significant results in retrospective studies."

Lesson

When you write your paper, do not only comment on the statistically significant changes that were found but also comment on if the results are clinically meaningful.

References

1. Bisla K, Tanelian DL. Concentration-dependent effects of *lidocaine* on corneal epithelial wound healing. Invest Ophthalmol Vis Sci. 1992;33:3029–33.
2. Wiggins WH, Zupfer GH, Jaffe RA, Angst AM, Brock-Utne JG. The addition of 5% glucose does not delay the onset of tourniquet pain for Bier block anesthesia. Anest Analg. 1998;86:S330.
3. Kain ZN. The legend of the P value (editorial). Anesth Analg. 2005;101:1454–6.
4. Simon R. Confidence intervals for reporting results of clinical trial. Ann Intern Med. 1986;105:429–35.
5. Feinstein AR. P values and confidence intervals: two sides of the same unsatisfactory coin. J Clin Epidemiol. 1998;51:355–60.
6. Gardner MG, Altman DG. Confidence intervals rather than P values: estimation rather than hypothesis testing. Br Med J. 1986;292:746–50.
7. Fisher RA. Statistical methods for research workers. 1st ed. Edinburgh: Oliver and Boyd, Reprinted by Oxford University Press; 1925.
8. Fisher RA. Design of experiments. 1st ed. Edinburgh: Oliver and Boyd, Reprinted by Oxford University Press; 1935.
9. Borenstein M. Hypothesis testing and effect size estimation in clinical trials. Ann Allergy Asthma Immunol. 1997;78:5–11.
10. Matthey S. P /0.05, but is it clinically significant? Practical examples for clinician. Behav Change. 1998;15:140–6.
11. Cummings P, Rivara FP. Reporting statistical information in medical journal articles. Arch Pediatr Adolesc Med. 2003;157:321–4.
12. Greenstein G. Clinical versus statistical significance as they relate to the efficacy of periodontal therapy. J AM Dent Assoc. 2003;134:583–91.
13. Sterne JAC, Smith GD, Cox D. Sifting the evidence: what's wrong with significance tests? Another comment on the role of statistical methods. Br Med J. 2001;322:226–31.
14. Kirk R. Practical significance: a concept whose time has come. Educ Psych Meas. 1996;56:746–59.
15. Snyder P, Lawson S. Evaluating results using corrected and uncorrected effect size estimates. J Exper Educ. 1993;61:334–49.
16. Greenberg RS, Bembea M, Heitmiller E. Rainy days for the society of pediatric anesthesia. Anesth Analg. 2012;114:1102–3.
17. Shafer SL, Dexter F. Publication bias, retrospective bias and reproducibility of significant results in observational studies. Anesth Analg. 2012;114:931–2.

Chapter 31
Case 31: How Many Authors?

You have, as the PI, completed a clinical study. Eight researchers participated. They include five clinicians, who obtained the consent from the patients and collected data; two physiologists, who reviewed the EEG tracings; and a statistician, who completed the statistical analysis. You choose an appropriate journal where you will send the manuscript. When you read the instructions to the author, you see that the journal allows only six authors and you have eight.

What would you do? Delete two authors; if so which ones? How do you approach the researchers whose names are to be deleted from the paper?

© Springer Science+Business Media New York 2015
J.G. Brock-Utne, *Clinical Research*, DOI 10.1007/978-1-4939-2516-2_31

Answer/Solution

1. You can write to the editor telling him/her you have a manuscript which you think will be suitable his/her journal, but you have eight authors. Would it be possible to make an exception? In my experience the editor will not.
2. Your only other option is to find another journal that is suitable and will take at least eight authors.
3. It is unacceptable to delete an author without any discussion (see Case 34).

Discussion

There is a perception that there are often too many authors on published papers. But multiauthored publications have become the norm. This is because research today is much more of a collaborative effort. With a team approach, you harness research expertise and save time and resources. Also private and/or federal funding organizations encourage collaboration and multidisciplinary projects.

Ben-Shlomo and Goodman [1] evaluated the number of authors from 1955 to 1985 in three journals (*Lancet*, *Circulation*, and *Fertility and Sterility*). There were 2–3 times more authors in 1985 as there were in 1955. The authors [1] conclude that the "active contribution by some participants (in the authorship of published articles) is reserved for the title, which alone bears the thumbprint of all." I agree with Grant [2] that this is "a sanctimonious campaign to stigmatize multiple authors of papers submitted to medical journals." Ben-Shlomo and Goodman imply that inclusion in the authors' list is often a gratuitous reward for some work done or for just being a "nice guy." Research training is and always has been a kind of apprenticeship, with younger workers learning the art of research from older more experienced researchers. It is a shame that authors like Ben-Shlomo and Goodman do not realize that the organization, execution, and write-up of even a minor clinical research project require a lot of time and effort. In 1955 and even in 1985, teamwork in research was rare. Today projects with the collaboration of other departments are common place. (Notice how Noble prizes in science are today very rarely given to a single person, but to a group of individuals, often from different universities and/or countries.) Most heads of departments in teaching hospitals surround themselves with a large number of scientifically motivated junior staff and research associates. Today projects are often based on a coordinated team effort. Research is no longer a cottage industry [3]. The techniques and equipment used are complicated and labor intensive. Very few of us have the skill to do everything, and hence there is a need for experts in the various fields. Multicenter trials and interdepartmental research necessitate an increase in the numbers of authors if the study is to be commenced and completed.

Epstein [4] confirmed the increased trend of multiple authorships and refers to the Vancouver convention [5]. Epstein mentions that the number has increased because of the "publish-or-perish" syndrome. However he feels that it is imperative that the trainee, who has contributed, be included in the final manuscript. This encourages "ownership," and maybe the person will be bitten by the research bug and become an academician. Not only should this trainee be included, but anyone who has contributed should have a say in the final product.

How do you decide who should be on the final paper? The best thing to do is to decide who should be on the authors' list and who should be first etc. at the very beginning of the study. You may change the order or add in others later, depending on their contribution. It is best that one person completes the first draft. Persons, who have simply given advice or technical assistance in the normal course of their work, should not be authors. Include only the head of the department and/or senior colleagues if they have contributed significantly to the paper. Never include anyone as an author without obtaining his or her approval. You should not cut anyone from the authors' list unless they request it. In the above example (Case 31), would you take out one of the physiologists who read the EEG or one of clinicians who worked tirelessly or the statistician who helped make the results meaningful?

An advisor should not have his/her name on the paper just because a researcher works in the advisor's laboratory. The advisor should be an author if he or she provides guidance, plays a central role in the ideas of the paper, participates in the discussion/execution of the paper, and helps prepare the final manuscript.

It can be difficult to establish the order in which the author's names should appear. As mentioned above, it is imperative to have the order established prior to the start of the study. There are no binding, universally agreed rules about this. I have always maintained that the author, who has contributed most to the successful conclusion of the work, should have his or her name first. If everyone has contributed equally, then one can arrange the names alphabetically or according to some convention that has been agreed to prior to the start of the study. It is well known that members of a team, who write several papers together, often take turns at being named as first author. If one person is clearly the catalyst to get the research going and concluded, then he or she is often either first or, if a senior author, last.

In a recent paper by Nylenna et al. [6] who studied the attitudes and practice of Norwegian researchers found the following: Almost all the researchers had knowledge of formal authorship requirements. Most of them agreed with the criteria, but found it hard to put them into practice. Interestingly, more experienced researchers found decisions on authorship and about the order of authors easier than less experienced researchers.

Lesson

Never delete an author in order to accommodate a journal's restriction on the number of authors. Find another journal if the editor won't allow the inclusion of all the authors.

References

1. Ben-Shlomo I, Goodman G. A place in the sun? Brit Med J. 1988;297:1631–2.
2. Grant IW. Multiple authorship. Brit Med J. 1989;298:386–7.
3. Rollin A-M. How many authors? (Ed). Anaesthesia. 1994;49:97–8.
4. Epstein RJ. Six authors in search of a citation: villains or victims of the Vancouver convention? Brit Med J. 1993;306:765–7.
5. International Committee of Medical Journal Editors Uniform requirements for manuscripts submitted to biomedical journals. Brit Med J. 1991;302:338–41
6. Nylenna M, Fagerbakk F, Kierulf P. Authorship: attitudes and practice among Norwegian researchers. BMC Med Ethics. 2014;15:53.

Chapter 32
Case 32: If You Injure Your Patient

We developed successfully in cats a neuromuscular rectal monitor to ascertain onset and recovery of neuromuscular drugs [1]. We thought it would be very useful in neonates and small children. This is because it is difficult to get reliable neuromuscular monitoring from a baby's small hand. Our devise consisted of an annular electrode (made of steel) and a transducing balloon.

After IRB approval and a mother's informed consent, we tested it out in a 6-month-old boy for exploratory laparotomy. The surgery and anesthesia went very well, but at the end of the surgery, we found that the baby had a large peritoneal burn. This was most probably caused by the small stainless steel ball that was part of the rectal monitor.

You do the following:

1. Inform the mother and apologize profusely.
2. Get the best treatment for the patient.
3. Stop the trial.
4. Inform the IRB about the problem that has occurred and tell them that you have stopped the trial.
5. Ask the IRB to stop the trial with immediate effect.
6. Tell the IRB that a full report will follow.

What else should you do?

© Springer Science+Business Media New York 2015
J.G. Brock-Utne, *Clinical Research*, DOI 10.1007/978-1-4939-2516-2_32

Answer/Solution

Publish this complication. It is imperative to warn the medical community about the problem that has occurred [2].

Discussion

The burn was caused by the electrical interaction between the diathermy and the stain steel head of the rectal probe. Luckily the child made an uneventful recovery.

Lesson

If you hurt a patient while doing your research, admit your error, get the best treatment, stop the trial, and warn the medical community of this problem.

References

1. Brock-Utne JG, Adam B, Downing JW. Monitoring neuromuscular blockade. Evaluation of a new rectal electrode/transducers system in cats. Anesth Analg. 1984;63:152–4.
2. Brock-Utne JG. Rectal monitor. Anesth Analg. 1984;63:1141.

Chapter 33
Case 33: Multicenter Trials

You, as an assistant professor, are invited to participate in a multicenter trial evaluating a new antiemetic. You are not aware of all the advantages and disadvantages of multicenter trials. But you do know that if you are the principal investigator (PI) in a multicenter trial, you have full control of the study execution and you will be the first author. It is well known that these trials generate a lot of research dollars. The funds go mainly to pay several research nurses to help do the study. The excess money is often used for other unfunded studies.

But what about if you are not the PI?

Are there any advantages for you, and what about disadvantages?

© Springer Science+Business Media New York 2015
J.G. Brock-Utne, *Clinical Research*, DOI 10.1007/978-1-4939-2516-2_33

Answer/Solution

There are very few advantages to you as an individual. But there is a big advantage to your department as it will get a large research fund. Your involvement may also help you to get promoted. However you should be aware of the many disadvantages. I will mention a few:

1. There is little benefit to you as a researcher. A nurse will do all the work. Your job will be just to check that the nurse is doing the study according to the protocol.
2. You will have very little or no input when the results and paper are written up. An example of no input is seen in the letter from Paul White [1]. In it he states that despite being a member of a multicenter trial, he was not given the opportunity to review the data or the manuscript before submission for publication to a peer-reviewed medical journal. Please also read the response by the authors who felt they adhered to all the principles of correct behavior [2]. Whatever side you take after reviewing these two letters, it is just unfortunate that they had to be published at all.
3. There will be no or very little input from you as to where and when the paper is published.
4. You will be one of over 20 authors, and if you are a junior investigator, you will be at the bottom of the authors' list, even if you have contributed over 200 of the 500 patients studied.
5. While the department will get paid in research dollars, most universities will take anything between 45 and 80 % to pay for their expenses. This takes the form of getting access to the hospital, paying the IRB, electricity, etc. If the university pays for the salaries of the research nurses, then they will take nearly 96 %.
6. It is difficult to find a strong and fair PI.
7. Often you have no choice as to the nurse or whoever else you must work with.
8. There is a lot of money involved. Each department is paid per case completed. Hence there are temptations to cut corners. In one study of pain medication for arthritic patients, over 50 % of the patients were later found not to have arthritis.

Another aspect of multicenter trials is that the sponsor often has control of the database. As Paul White [1] states and I quote: "…this type of action raises a serious question as to transparency of a multicenter study, where the database is completely controlled by the sponsor" [1]. There are many publications raising several issues regarding potential conflict of interest and industry involvement in peer-reviewed publications [3–8].

Lesson

Multicenter trials have very little benefit to you as a researcher, unless you are the PI. The university may of course thank you for raising a lot of money for them. It may also help you in getting promoted.

References

1. White PF. The importance of transparency in industry-sponsored multicenter clinical studies. Anesth Analg. 2007;105:1861.
2. Gan TJ, Apfel CC, Kovac A, Philip BK, Singla N, Minkowitz H, Habib AS, Carides A, Horgan KJ, Evans JK, Lawsson FC. The importance of transparency in industry-sponsored multicenter clinical studies. Anesth Analg. 2007;105:1861–2.
3. Saidman LJ. Unresolved issues relating to peer review, industry support of research, and conflict of interest. Anesthesiology. 1994;80:491–2.
4. Peterson FJ. Industry support of research and conflict of interest. Anesthesiology. 1994;81:270.
5. Eger EI. Motivation, bias and scientific integrity. Anesthesiology. 1994;81:270–1.
6. Davidoff F, DeAngelis CD, Drazen JM, Hoey J, Hojgaard L, Horton R, Nicholls MG, Nylenna M, Overbeke AJ, Sox HC, Van Der Weyden MB, Wilkes MS. Sponsorship, authorship and accountability. Lancet. 2001;358:854–6.
7. Brennan TA, Rothman DJ, Blank L, Blumenthal D, Chimonas SC, Cohen JJ, Goldman J, Kassirer JP, Kimball H, Naughton J, Smelser N. Health industry practices that create conflicts of interest: a policy proposal for academic medical centers. JAMA. 2006;295:429–33.
8. Newcombe JP, Kerridge IH. Assessment of human research ethics committees of potential conflicts of interest arising from pharmaceutical sponsorship of clinical research. Intern Med J. 2007;37:12–7.

Chapter 34
Case 34: Unprofessional Behavior

You have participated in a clinical study. Your role has been very active, as you have helped produce the protocol and the consent form and got it passed by the IRB. You made data sheets and collected some of the patient's data. You even helped write up the paper. However when the paper is finally published, you discover that your name is not on it.

What will you do?

© Springer Science+Business Media New York 2015

J.G. Brock-Utne, *Clinical Research*, DOI 10.1007/978-1-4939-2516-2_34

Answer/Solution

This happened to me. I discovered that there was very little I could do to remedy this unprofessional behavior. What I did was to write to all the authors asking for an explanation. I heard nothing in writing, but the first author rang me and told me it was not his fault. He said that the editor was at fault, as he had not allowed seven authors on the paper. The maximum for that journal was six. The first author told me that he had spoken to the editor and was assured that all seven would be included. When checking with the editor, I was told that no such arrangement had been requested, nor would it have been accepted. If you need the paper added to your curriculum vitae, you could write to the Dean of the Medical School and ask him to do so. I did not do that.

Discussion

It can be a difficult task to be a PI in charge of a collaborate study. He or she must build trust and collegiality. Every member of the team must understand the study's aim and each participant's role. It is imperative to delineate the roles and responsibilities of each member. Fairness and accountability must be developed. If not, then the collaboration will suffer. There can be disagreements, about how the study should be done, who the authors should be and the order, who is responsible for the data, how to handle problems when there is evidence of lack of compliance, etc.

As mentioned in Case 31, the problem of who should be first author can be difficult. This should preferably be done before the study starts. Usually the first author is the one who has contributed the most. Many senior authors, although they have done a considerable amount of work, give the first author status to a junior member of the team, thereby hoping to advance the junior researcher's career.

Lesson

If you have done a considerable amount of work for a study but get omitted from the author's list, then my advice is do nothing and have nothing more to do with these coworkers.

Chapter 35
Case 35: Tips on How to Get the Institutional Review Board (IRB) Submission Completed and Passed

You must have an IRB approval to do clinical research, even if it consist of something as simple and risk-free as noninvasively taking the patient's pulse. Although a study which consists of just taking the patient's pulse is not considered a risk to the subject, informed consent is required. If you are unsure of whether you need informed consent, always contact your local IRB.

The most important part of the IRB submission is the informed consent.

What are the tips that will make:

1. The informed consent easy for both the IRB panel and a potential research subject to understand?
2. Potential research subjects wanting to participate in a study?

© Springer Science+Business Media New York 2015
J.G. Brock-Utne, *Clinical Research*, DOI 10.1007/978-1-4939-2516-2_35

Answer/Solution

Informed consent must:

1. Be short, simple, and understandable for a 14-year-old (a grade 8 reading level). In developing countries, the informed consent form must be appropriately tailored to make sure people are properly informed before signing on. The World health organization-council for international organizations of medical sciences (WHO-CIOMS) guidelines state: "Ideally, each potential research subject should possess the intellectual capacity and insight to provide valid informed consent, and enjoy the independence to exercise absolute freedom of choice over the extent of collaboration without fear of discrimination. However, many investigations, and particularly those intended to serve the interests of under privileged communities and vulnerable minorities including children and the mentally ill, would be debarred if the preconditions were accepted as mandatory criteria for recruitment."
2. Be explained in detail by the researcher to the intended research subject.
3. Not contain difficult words.
4. Be signed prior to the start with a date and a witness signature.
5. Include a separate information sheet about the Health Insurance Portability Accountability Act (HIPAA) that also must be signed, dated, and witnessed.

Furthermore if the patient seems unsure/unhappy/confused/worried/angry/belligerent/irritated about participating in the study, then don't let them sign on to the study. Never manipulate or gently force anyone to be part of anything they don't want to do. If anything goes wrong (see Case 32) and you are perceived to have manipulated the patient to participate, this could be a major problem.

Discussion

There are at least two safeguards that are required prior to enrolling a subject in a clinical trial. Firstly there is an independent committee (IRB) which does both a scientific and ethical review of the proposal. The committee is independent and has a diverse membership. Secondly the voluntary consent of the subject must be given prior to the study [1].

It is imperative that a study is not exposing a subject to a significant risk. To do a study at the expense of the overall well-being of a subject is not acceptable. The IRB is there to help minimize the risk to the participants. Before you submit your proposal, always ask yourself the following questions:

1. Does the risk to the subject outweigh the potential benefit to that subject?
2. Would you like your mother to participate in this study?
3. Is the study designed well enough to give valid answers to the questions posed? Does the study warrant the expenditure of time and effort?

If you are happy with your answers, then proceed with the IRB submission. Otherwise suggest another way to study the clinical problem.

IRB in the USA was established by the Research Act of 1974 (under Title 45 CFR Part 46). It is regulated by the FDA and each individual hospital policy. The IRB has usually five members, with enough experience, expertise, and diversity to render an unbiased opinion. The committee must consist of one scientist, a nonscientist, a community member, and a lawyer who should be a vulnerable population advocate. Men and woman should both be present. At present most institutions require that their researchers do the Collaborative Institutional Training Initiative (CITI). This is a web-based training program with different modules like IRB regulations, informed consent, genetic research, vulnerable subjects, history and ethical principles, patient privacy and confidentiality, and monitoring safety. Many institutions now require you to take these modules before you can submit an IRB application.

The definition of research (Department of Health and Human Services in the Code of Federal Regulations (45 CFR 46. 102(d))) is defined as "The systematic investigation, including research development, testing and evaluation, designed to develop or contribute to generalizable knowledge." The definition can be interpreted in several ways so another human research definition has been proposed (45CFR 46. 102 (f)): "The definition of a human subject is a living individual about whom an investigator (whether professional or student) conducting research, obtains [1] data through intervention or interaction with the individual or [2] identifiable private information."

Since I started doing clinical research in 1968, the regulatory burden for the clinical researcher has increased enormously. This can be seen in our recent letter to the editor [2]. The letter dealt with a resubmitted in 2010, of a 1990 research protocol. The 1990 study involved a new noninvasive blood pressure monitor. The blood pressure result from this monitor was compared to values obtained from an invasive radial arterial line in the same patient. After approval in 1990, the study was completed and published [3]. Although the protocol submitted in 2010 was identical to the one submitted in 1990, the length of the required consent form increased from two and half pages to eight pages. The word count increased from 689 to 2,596. The increase was mainly due to the additional information requirements pertaining to HIPAA (Health Insurance Portability and Accountability Act), the Experimental Subject's Bill of Rights, and the wording which pertains to the notification of risk and compensation for research-related injuries.

In our submission [2], we concluded that the IRB's overly conservative approach is designed mainly to protect the institution and not necessarily to improve the safety of the research subjects. The enlarged consent form has in our opinion not added to patient safety, but rather increased the anxiety for the patient.

Lesson

IRB submission has become unnecessarily complicated and time consuming. But there is little you can do about it. My best advice is to answer the questions on the form as simply, clearly, and concisely as you can.

References

1. Denham JE, Nelson RM. Self-determination is not an appropriate model for understanding parental permission and child assent. Anesth Analg. 2002;94:1049–51.
2. Esaki R, Macario A, Harrison TK, Brock-Utne JG. The IRB process needs to be re-examined. Anesth Analg. 2011;112:1249.
3. Siegel LC, Brock-Utne JG, Brodsky JB. Comparison of arterial tonometry with radial Artery catheter measurements of blood pressure in anesthetized patients. Anesthesiology. 1994;81:578–84.

Chapter 36
Case 36: How to Perform and Report the Result of a Survey

A resident seeks help from you with a survey he/she wants to send out to all the medical residents in training programs in the Western United States. The survey relates to working conditions, housing, research time, study time, travel to and from hospitals etc.

There is no doubt that surveys are becoming increasingly used in our personal and professional lives. But many times the conclusion from the survey may be questionable.

What are the facts that you must keep in mind when advising someone on how to construct a survey?

© Springer Science+Business Media New York 2015   91
J.G. Brock-Utne, *Clinical Research*, DOI 10.1007/978-1-4939-2516-2_36

Answer/Solution

There are many facts as can be seen below.

Discussion

The excellent editorial by Burmeister [1] has been very valuable in answering this question. I have added my own comments in point form below:

1. For a valid result of a survey, it is important to define who are to be surveyed. In this case it is medical residents. It is also important to differentiate each individual by age, sex, place of work, specialty, and stage reached in their educational training. The residents at the beginning of their training may have very different views of the working conditions than their more senior colleagues. The lists of residents from each institution must be current so that all eligible participants are given an opportunity to fill in the survey. If the above recommendations are not adhered to, the survey may be biased and/or inaccurate. Burmeister [1] states that the result of a survey given to people twice with 2-year interval gave very different results.

2. You are well advised to copy a well-researched and published survey. However if some of your questions are new or different, you should do a pilot study to evaluate comments to those questions.

3. There is no easy way to determine what constitutes an adequate sample size when dealing with a survey. A sample size is, according to Burmeister [1], not selecting a specific percentage of the residents, but rather looking at "the desired precision of characteristics to be estimated and the confidence level assigned to achieve this specified precision." If a theory is to be tested, it is essential to increase the sample size because statistical power is an additional consideration. It may be necessary to stratify the results by age and/or experience. This should improve the precisions and even reduce the necessary sample size for a specified level of precisions. Remember that using the cluster sampling will most likely also decrease the precision. If one elects to use both stratified and cluster sampling techniques, then the analysis may require a computer program such a SUDAAN (Survey Data Analysis). Without using the SUDAAN in such a survey, the results may prove misleading.

4. It is imperative to note the number of nonresponders. Obviously the results from a 30 % participation may be very different from one with 50 % participation, leading to misleading results. Burmeister states that "Nonresponse bias is equal to the proportion of nonresponse multiplied by the difference of the responders and non-responders; consequently, there is no absolutely level of response." Nuttall et al. [2], who published a survey done by the American Society of Anesthesiologists Committee on transfusion medicine, clearly increased the initial sample size to accommodate a relatively low expected response rate.

Increasing the sample size does not eliminate nonresponse bias. What should have been done was "to decrease the initial sample size and increase the efforts to contact the initial non-responders" [1].

5. There will always be some who will not complete a survey no matter how simple or short it is. Nonresponders have their own reason for not participating which rank from "no time/could not be bothered" to "not wanting their opinions noted." The latter relates to their belief that the survey is not blinded. It is virtually impossible to eliminate nonresponse bias in these types of surveys. Hence it is essential to describe the potential nonresponse bias and minimize the fraction of nonresponders. By providing the demographics of the studied population, the bias of nonresponders will be minimized. It is a fact that nearly even demographic characteristics cannot rule out potential nonresponse bias. A second attempt to contact nonresponders may increase some participation, but there are studies to show that two attempts at the same survey do not necessarily give the same response.

6. Incentives and endorsements, from heads of all the departments that are participating in the study, may improve the number of participants. But these efforts will not eliminate a nonresponse bias.

Lesson

It is important in surveys like this to make every effort to reduce the proportion of nonresponders. Burmeister [1] recommends that every effort must be made to sample all nonresponders.

Surveys are important research tools, but they are challenging to carry out. As can be seen from the above, it has inherent limitation. But that should not prevent a potential researcher from attempting to do a survey. This is because surveys can make important contribution to patient care and our performance as clinicians.

References

1. Burmeister LF. Principles of successful sample surveys. Anesthesiology. 2003;99:125–52.
2. Nuttall GA, Stehling LC, Beighley CM, Faust RJ. American Society of Anesthesiologist committee on transfusion medicine: current transfusion practices of members of the American Society of Anesthesiologists. A survey. Anesthesiology. 2003;99:1433–43.

Chapter 37
Case 37: Validity of the Cricoid Pressure (Sellick's Maneuver)

A young assistant professor approaches you with a suggestion for a clinical study. He has entitled it:

"The validation of the cricoid pressure (CP)."

He states that there has been a lack of studies to show that the maneuver prevents passive regurgitation. He quotes two systematic reviews that conclude that there is no evidence either for or against the maneuver [1, 2].

He is interested in doing a study to attempt to:

1. Answer the question: Is properly applied cricoid pressure effective in preventing regurgitation?
2. Validate the efficacy of cricoid pressure in reducing the incidence of pulmonary aspiration.

What will you tell him?

© Springer Science+Business Media New York 2015
J.G. Brock-Utne, *Clinical Research*, DOI 10.1007/978-1-4939-2516-2_37

Answer/Solution

1. By looking at Sellick's original data, he could find out how many subjects is needed per group [3]. Fifty subjects per group are needed to prove that CP is ten times more effective than no pressure to reduce the incidence of passive regurgitation from 12 to 1.2 % (alpha 1, 0.05 and beta, 0.2) [3, 4]. He then should do a randomized trial.
2. This is a much more difficult study, i.e., to test whether CP reduces the incidence of pulmonary aspiration. This will require a much larger sample size. If one considers the frequency of aspiration to be approximately 0.15 % in adults, a randomized trial to reduce the incidence of aspiration by 50 % would require a sample size of 25,000 patients in each group. This is an unacceptable sample size, and furthermore I doubt that it would be passed by any IRB. If the study was passed, then it should be done as a large multicenter trial to have any chance of finishing it in 1 year.

Discussion

That leaves only option 1 which is suggested by Lerman [4]. However I doubt that this study would be passed by an IRB. There is also the question of which patient population to study. Would the patients have a trauma and/or bowel obstruction etc.? What preoperative medication should be given like antacid, metoclopramide, narcotics, etc.? Are you going to attempt to empty the stomach preoperatively or not? There is also the question of what constitutes a properly applied CP?

It would be imperative to establish the amount of gastric fluid present preoperatively prior to a rapid sequence induction and intubation (RSII). Then hopefully one can establish if CP may be effective when, for example, there is 100 mL of gastric fluid present at preinduction. Let's say the study is approved and starts and you discover a study patient that has over 500 mL of gastric juice present preinduction. Then it would not be ethical not to do everything you can (gastric or nasogastric tube, CP, Bicitra, and metoclopramide) to prevent aspiration. There is no doubt that the result of a validation of CP will be important to the practicing physician, be it an anesthesiologist, an emergency physician, or an ICU physician. Unfortunately for all the reasons listed above, this study will not be done. This means that we must carry on using CP even though there is no real proof of its efficacy. It is worth bearing in mind that judges and juries have ruled against anesthesiologists who did not apply CP, both in the USA and UK [4]. In the USA, on average, if an anesthesiologist is found guilty and has not used CP, then the payout to the patient is twice as much as if CP had been performed.

It is interesting to note that in a study, 4 % ($n = 12$) had evidence of new or unexpected chest infiltrate on chest X-rays after endotracheal intubation. This is despite the fact that nine had CP during RSII [5]. Fenton and Reynolds [6] reviewed the results of nearly 5,000 general anesthetics for obstetrical surgery in Malawi. Eleven deaths were attributed to regurgitation and nine had CP applied. As Lerman [4] states, these studies and other smaller studies with similar results do not bode well for proving that CP is effective in preventing poor outcomes [7, 8].

Lesson

In my opinion, the study to validate cricoid pressure, although worthwhile, will never be done. Hence the physician has to carry out gastric emptying (mechanically or with drugs), increase the lower esophageal sphincter tone [9], and use properly applied CP [10] in the hope that aspiration does not occur.

References

1. Neilipovitz DT, Crosby ET. No evidence for decreased incidence of aspiration after rapid sequence induction. Can J Anaesth. 2007;54:748–64.
2. Brimacombe JR, Berry AM. Cricoid pressure. Can J Anaesth. 1997;44:414–25.
3. Sellick BA. Cricoid pressure to prevent regurgitation of stomach contents during induction of anesthesia. Lancet. 1961;278:404–6.
4. Lerman J. On cricoid pressure: "may the force be with you" (Ed). Anesth Anal. 2009;109:1363–6.
5. Schwartz DE, Matthey MA, Cohen NH. Death and other complications of emergency airway management in critically ill adults a prospective investigations of 297 tracheal intubations. Anesthesiology. 1995;82:367–76.
6. Fenton PM, Reynolds F. Life-savings or ineffective? An observational study of the use of cricoid pressure and maternal outcome in an African setting. Int J Obstet Anesth. 2009;18:106–10.
7. Whittington RM, Robinson JS, Thompson JM. Fatal aspiration (Mendelson's) syndrome despite antacids and cricoid pressure. Lancet. 1979;31:228–30.
8. Williamson R. Cricoid pressure (letter). Can J Anaesth. 1989;36:601.
9. Brock-Utne JG, Downing JW. The lower oesophageal sphincter (LOS) and the anaesthetist. S Afr Med J. 1986;70:170–1.
10. Brock-Utne JG. Is cricoid pressure necessary? (Ed). Paediatr Anaesth. 2002;12:1–4.

Chapter 38
Case 38: Another Unprofessional Behavior

A colleague (Dr. X) participated in a clinical study. His involvement consisted of obtaining informed consent from the patients and collecting data and blood samples from about 1/3 of the 60 patients in the trial. The study was concluded. There were five authors. The draft manuscript was circulated around for all the authors to review. Dr. X strongly disagrees with the way the methodology section was written. He stated that the study was not randomized. Since the other four think that it was randomized and will not concede, Dr. X withdrew from the authors list.

Nine months later, he found that the paper was published in the Lancet, without his name, but in his opinion describing the wrong "methodology."

He wrote to the editor claiming academic "fraud." The letter was published, but the other four authors did not get an offer to respond. After the four authors read the letter in the journal, a heated argument ensued between Dr. X and the authors of the paper. The Dean, the Principal, and the Ombudsman of the university became involved in the impasse.

If you were Dr. X what would you have done?

© Springer Science+Business Media New York 2015
J.G. Brock-Utne, *Clinical Research*, DOI 10.1007/978-1-4939-2516-2_38

Answer/Solution

Dr. X should have:

1. Removed all his data sheets and after that refused to discuss the project any further
2. Not written to the editor

Discussion

You don't do research to become famous and wealthy, especially at the expense of others. Sadly at academic centers, envy can occur and feuds develop, which often last for years. Evidence of these feuds can be seen in the "Letter to Editor" sections of many journals. The editor's responsibility here is enormous.

Research should foster friendships, not enemies. (The latter is counterproductive for everyone involved.) Remember Francois Rabelais (1492–1553), a major French Renaissance writer, doctor, and Renaissance humanist, who said: "Science with conscience is the soul's perdition" or "Science without conscience is the ruin of the soul."

In the above case, it is interesting to note that all five authors left the university within 1 year.

Lesson

If you feel that your other coworkers are not honorable, it is not worth leaving your name on the paper, even if you have done a lot of the work. The best thing to do is to remove all your data sheets, consent forms, and withdraw from the project.

Chapter 39
Case 39: A Dataset

You are a new assistant professor in a medical department in a large university hospital. An associate professor is leaving the department the day you arrive. He hands you a dataset of 140 patients with chronic obstructive lung disease (COPD). The dataset contains variables which he has collected. They vary from sex, age, address, BMI, race, presence of hair, hair color, alcohol use, past surgical history, smoking history, drug treatments, family history of COPD, hypertension, etc. He asks you to analyze the data and submit the results as an abstract to the next annual meeting of respiratory diseases. He just wants to be second author. After that you don't see him again.

You enter all the data into a multiple regression model. Statistical significant findings are shown between severity of COPD and BMI, which is understandable. However many different significances are found between severity of COPD and a blood group, address, eye color, etc.

You submit the abstract with the association only between COPD and BMI. You elect to omit the other significant associations as you can't understand or explain them.

Is this the correct way of reporting the results or should all the other associations have been included, even if you can't explain them?

Answer/Solution

You must have a hypothesis PRIOR to examining the patient data. Our assistant professor should have asked the associate professor what was the question or hypothesis he wanted to elucidate.

The correct way would have been to use the data to generate a hypothesis and then validate it with another set of observations. After the second set of observations, one could draw a more definite conclusion. Remember you can't use the same data again to generate or test the hypothesis.

It is important to realize that an association between two or more variables may be the result of a chance difference in the distribution of these variables. I will always remember a Scandinavian medical meeting held in Stockholm in the 1970s. A large dataset was analyzed and showed a lot of statistically significant associations. The speaker told the audience that these associations were scientifically valid results despite the fact that he had not done another set of observations. At the end of the presentation, an old and wise Swedish professor stood up and said: "I am sure that you are aware that it is a statistically significant fact that the birthrate in southern Sweden increases with the influx of storks." He then sat down to a thundering applause.

Andersen [1] states correctly that without hypothesis generating activities, there would be no hypothesis to test and clinical research would be without purpose.

Lesson

Hypothesis testing is essential in clinical research. But it is imperative to have a hypothesis prior to analyzing any data. If not, you will get a lot of associations that may not be relevant unless you collect a second set of data.

Reference

1. Andersen B. Methodological errors in medical research. Oxford: Blackwell; 1990.

Suggested Reading

Supino PG, Borer JS, editors. Principles of research methodology, A guide for clinical investigators. New York: Springer; 2012.

Chapter 40
Case 40: Taking Over an Ongoing Clinical Trial

You have been put in charge of a clinical laboratory in a university hospital. A long-term clinical study is ongoing which you are now in charge of. There is a massive amount of data being generated. You are fully aware of the hypothesis and understand the questions that are being posed. A nurse coordinator is in charge of the handling and storage of data, while a senior technician is in charge of analyzing and reporting on it.

A few days after you take over, both the nurse coordinator and the senior technician resign.

What questions should you ask them about the study before they leave?

© Springer Science+Business Media New York 2015
J.G. Brock-Utne, *Clinical Research*, DOI 10.1007/978-1-4939-2516-2_40

Answer/Solution

I list some of the questions in no particular order:

1. Is the study supported by a grant? If so, when was it last renewed and when is it to be renewed again?
2. What information does the granting body require for renewal and is the study up to date in this regard?
3. How is the data stored and handled?
4. How is the data communicated to the technician? Does he have all the data? Or have there been incidences when data was lost?
5. When is the IRB coming up for renewal?
6. How many study patients have been completed and how many are left?
7. Does the nurse think that the study will be finished prior to the study's IRB expiration? If not, do we have all the information needed to apply for an extension of the IRB (number of patients studied, sex, and ages)?
8. Has the statistical power to confirm the hypotheses been done?
9. Are there any problems which make it impossible/difficult to complete the study? Are other departments needed to complete the study? Are they cooperating? Are they involved as authors or not?
10. How many patients had to be excluded to date and why?
11. Are there any concerns about obtaining informed consent? What is the success rate?
12. Is there any possibility that the study may not be completed on time? If so, why?
13. What does the financial balance sheet of the project look like? Are new grants expected? Are there enough finances to finish the study?

You are asking these questions to try to find any evidence of poor research planning that may hinder the successful completion of the data collection. If there is poor planning then you must try and rectify it—if possible.

Lesson

Taking over an ongoing research project is fraught with dangers. This is not the time to take anything for granted. Check your facts. You will never regret it.

Chapter 41
Case 41: Should You Do a Pilot Study in This Proposed Trial?

An evaluation of an outpatient education program was proposed and designed by a senior member of staff. You, as a junior academic member of the department, are put in charge of this 2-year study. The trial involves four hospitals in the same district. Patients with chronic bowel disorders are enrolled with their informed consent. In two hospitals, the patients are given a new educational program related to their disease, administered by a nurse coordinator. In the other two hospitals, the patients are not given a program. All patients are given two depression and anxiety tests. In the group that gets the educational program, the tests will be a pre- and post assessment. This is to ascertain any change in their depression and anxiety.

You have the following concerns with the proposed trial:

1. The two scales that have been chosen to assess the depression and anxiety have not been tested in this population group. You consult a psychologist who said there would be concerns about the validity of the tests and accordingly the results.
2. Who will train the nurse coordinator to present the educational program?
3. One hospital in the test group has a very different social economic group of patients compared to the other three. You wonder if this is of concern and are told it is not.

Based on the above, you suggest a pilot study. However, the senior member states that this is unnecessary as it will be in his opinion, both a waste of time and subjects.

How will you respond? Forgo the pilot study or proceed with it?

© Springer Science+Business Media New York 2015
J.G. Brock-Utne, *Clinical Research*, DOI 10.1007/978-1-4939-2516-2_41

Answer/Solution

Insist on a pilot study.

Discussion

Faced with this sort of problem, always insist on a pilot study. This is despite the fact that you will probably become unpopular with one or more departmental members. If members are unhappy, it is a very good idea to invite all the members of the department to a 1-h research discussion on the proposed study. Do remember to bring in your expert like, in this case, the psychologist.

If you have to do the study without a pilot trial, then you must insist on an interim analysis after 6 months. This will cost time and effort, but should be done.

Also, never forget to educate the nurse coordinator on what is to be taught. You must check and record any interventions. The training of the nurse will take time, but is imperative to do it. This would be especially true in the example above, because of the big difference between the social economic groups in two test hospitals. Educational intervention must always take into account the educational background of the patients.

If the study in this example is completed, it will most likely not be published as your concerns (1,2,3) will be easily recognized by most reviewers of peer-reviewed journals. Similar studies are often not published, as they are considered either incomplete, the material not comparable, the methodology not appropriate, and/or do not reach statistical significance.

Always remember to do a pilot study, especially when there are complexities with the patient population, questionable methodology, concerns over collection procedures, etc. If the pilot trial is successful, then it may be used to obtain funding. If it is unsuccessful, then you can either abandon the present plan or modify the plan by altering the study design. Should the pilot trial indicate that the study will take too much time, then you can modify the question, broaden the inclusion criteria, add additional study sites, relax the exclusion criteria, alter the study design, etc.

The book by Marks [1] is well worth reading as he has several vignettes to show how poor research planning can lead to non-publishable results. He states: "The success of a research project depends on how well thought out a project is and how potential problems have been identified and resolved before data collection begins."

Lesson

Research planning is essential for a successful trial. If a pilot study is indicated, do it.

Reference

1. Mark RG. Designing a research project. The basics of biomedical research methodology. Belmont: Lifetime. Learning Publications: A division of Wadsworth; 1982

Chapter 42
Case 42: An Inconclusive Result (Negative Result): What to Do

You have just completed a clinical study in volunteers. The study attempted to evaluate the respiratory depression of two drugs by using the CO_2 response curve. One group received morphine and the other group diazepam, given in two different doses intravenously. You are surprised to see that the study shows no difference between the two groups of volunteers.

Your senior coworker suggests that this inconclusive (negative) result will be of no interest to any journal and you are wasting your time submitting it.

What will you do and what can you do to improve your chances of getting it published?

© Springer Science+Business Media New York 2015   109
J.G. Brock-Utne, *Clinical Research*, DOI 10.1007/978-1-4939-2516-2_42

Answer/Solution

Always attempt to submit, even if the study is inconclusive, does not support the hypothesis, etc. You have put too much effort into it not to submit it. Also you may feel, like I feel, that all clinical trials, if done appropriately, should be published. The main reason is that negative results could save time and money for another researcher who is considering embarking on a similar study.

Discussion

To improve your chances of a publication of a negative study, it must first have been adequately powered and well designed. We are told that this is not the case with most inconclusive studies [1].

Many years ago Dr. Mannie Mankowitz, John W. Downing, and I completed such a study. It was adequately powered and we thought the paper addressed an important clinical question. After submitting it to five journals and receiving no acceptance, I put it in my filing cabinet, where it is still lying. I know it will remain there. But it is difficult to throw it out, as it was a lot of work. It is called the "file drawer effect." My senior colleague (JWD) was correct in telling me that my attempt of getting it published was a waste of time.

It is a fact that premiere medical journals are far more likely to publish positive results rather than negative findings [2, 3]. This phenomenon is known as a publication bias [2, 3]. However one editor states that he makes an effort to publish negative results provided they are adequately powered and address an important clinical question [4]. However other editors will say [1] that studies with a negative primary result do not resolve the research question. Therefore when reading a negative results paper, one must be very cautious about interpreting the findings. Also many authors do not submit studies with negative results. But I believe a study showing negative or no results can be illuminating.

For your information there are journals that specialize in negative results, they include:

1. Journal of Negative Results (URL:http://www.jnr-eeb.org/index.php/jnr)
2. Journal of Negative Results in BioMedicine (URL:http://www.jnrbm.com)
3. Journal of Pharmaceutical Negative Results (URL:http://www.pnrjournal.com)
4. Journal of Articles in Support of the Null Hypothesis (URL:http://www.jasnh.com)

If you do submit a paper with negative result, don't indicate that your study failed and therefore was a waste of time. Rather say something like this: "The way the study was done could not reject the null hypothesis and therefore we caution other researchers about using this methodology." In other words, you are informing your colleagues what not to do.

Lesson

If the result of a completed study, which was adequately powered and addressed an important clinical question, was inconclusive, then you must always seek publication.

References

1. Houle T. Negative studies scarce in anesthesia journals. Anesthesiol News. 2011;10–3
2. De Oliveira Jr GS, Chang R, Kendall MC, Fitzgerald PC, McCarthy RJ. Publication bias in anesthesiology literature. Anesth Analg. 2012;114:1042–8.
3. Easterbrook PJ, Berlin JA, Gopalan R, Matthews DR. Publication bias in clinical research. Lancet. 1991;337:867–72.
4. Shafer SL. Negative studies scarce in anesthesia journals. Anesthesiol News. 2011;10–3

Chapter 43
Case 43: Retrospective Studies: What to Watch Out For

You are an Associate Professor in a large university hospital. An anesthesia resident asks you if it is possible to use the large hospital database to attempt to answer a clinical question. The question relates to the prediction of hypotension after induction of general anesthesia. He suggests that all episodes of post-induction hypotension be extracted from the database and the associated factors be analyzed.

He asks if:

1. He needs an IRB approval for the database chart review?
2. He needs a written protocol and/or research plan?
3. This is an important question?
4. You have any thoughts about retrospective studies, as he has heard negative comments about them?

What is your reply?

© Springer Science+Business Media New York 2015   113
J.G. Brock-Utne, *Clinical Research*, DOI 10.1007/978-1-4939-2516-2_43

Answer/Solution

1. You tell him to ask the IRB if a chart review in this case could be "IRB exempt." It is most likely that the chart review will be IRB exempt if the chart review is done using "de-identified" anonymous data. If the database cannot produce "de-identified" anonymous data, then an IRB approval must be sought.

2. A written research plan is mandatory so as to conceptualize the study. As mentioned before, it is essential to have adequate planning if you are to achieve your research objectives. In this case, it is important to identify the independent associations leading to hypotension, for instance, drug doses, how sick the patient is, etc.

3. You tell him that his proposed study may be good for an abstract at a resident and/or annual society conference. If it is adequately powered, it may be accepted in a peer-review journal as there are examples of that in the literature [1–4].

   You tell him also that, if he was to embark on this study, he should seek statistical help, so the study is not unpowered. He must also have a definition of hypotension in mmHg.

4. There are inherent problems with all retrospective studies, ranging from data entry to biases, both known and unknown. There is also a lack of control, which prevents an evaluation of cause and effect. Silbert et al. [5] state that even the very best conducted retrospective studies can provide level 3 evidence only. Usually results of retrospective studies indicate a need for prospective randomized controlled trials [6].

This retrospective study will not answer what predicts hypotension directly. The question of how relevant a short episode of hypotension could be is not addressed either.

Schonberger [7] warns of distortion effects stemming from imperfect comorbidity coding. Take for an example that anesthesiologists in the university hospital where you work, as an associate professor, prefer to use nitrous oxide in health patients and not in sicker patients. This fact could therefore distort an observed odds ratio compared to the actual odds ratio which is present between samples. Schonberger [7] states: "The supposition that nonbiased, random errors in ascertaining outcomes will not affect observed odds ratios between sample populations is a common misperception."

Lesson

Retrospective studies have inherited problems that must always be born in mind. An IRB exempt or approval must be sought. A written research plan and a presentation to your peers to get sufficient feedback are imperative. If you do embark on such a study, make sure that the study is not unpowered and the groups are comparable.

References

1. Luce V, Auoy Y, Benhamou D. What good are large databases of intraoperative data? Anesth Analg. 2006;103:251.
2. Reich DL, Hossain S, Krol M, et al. Predictors of hypotension after induction of general anesthesia. Anesth Analg. 2004;23:788–93.
3. Fasting S, Gisvold SE. Data recording of problems during anaesthesia: presentation of a well functioning and simple system. Acta Anaesthesiol Scan. 1996;40:1173–83.
4. Tremper KK. Anesthesia information systems: developing the physiologic phenotype database. Anesth Analg. 2005;101:620–1.
5. Silbert BS, Evered LA, Scott DA. Cognitive decline after surgery and illness. Anesthesiology. 2010;112:1182–4.
6. Silverstein JH, Allore HG, Deiner S, Sano M, Rasmussen L. Is postoperative cognitive decline clinically relevant? Anesthesiology. 2010;112:1280–1.
7. Schonberger RB. Random errors and misclassification bias. Analg Anesth. 2014;119:497–8.

Chapter 44
Case 44: Plagiarism

You have just completed a clinical study with a resident. You ask him to write the first draft. He finishes the draft and hands it to you after 2 weeks. You read it through, but are concerned that there are parts, both in the methodology and the discussion, which you think are plagiarized from previous texts. You check and discover that you are correct.

Plagiarism is misconduct. Remember what Marcel C. LaFolette (1910–1955), a research associate at the Smithsonian Institution in Washington, DC, said: "Forgery, fakery and plagiarism contradict every natural expectation for how scientists act: they challenge every positive image of science that society holds."

You call the resident to your office. He understands that plagiarism is not appropriate, but he asks you if there a difference between plagiarism of a description of a method and plagiarism of what is written in the discussion and/or introduction.

What is your response?

© Springer Science+Business Media New York 2015
J.G. Brock-Utne, *Clinical Research*, DOI 10.1007/978-1-4939-2516-2_44

Answer/Solution

A description of a method is not considered plagiarism if the method used in the submitted manuscript is identical to what has been described before [1]. If you change the wordings in a methodology and not reference the method, then the reviewer may suspect/worry that you have not used the prescribed methodology. If published and not corrected, the reader could also be concerned/confused.

Discussion

Plagiarism of discussions and/or introductions is not appropriate (see Case 22). The editor today utilizes a software program to identify plagiarism [2]. Mazoit [3] states that such software like CrossCheck makes it more difficult for non-English-speaking/writing researchers to write a paper in English and submit it to an English journal. One solution for non-English writers is to submit the paper to a journal in their own country first. However, there may not be one that is suitable. If a non-English-speaking researcher gets his work published in his/her language, then he/she can submit it to an English journal. However it is imperative that the author discloses any prior publication, outlining the same results. They may also have to provide a written consent from the holder of the copyright. Dr. Shafer [2] states: "If this is not done, then unfortunately the second publication represents a duplicate publication, and is also a copyright violation (at least under United States law)."

Another example of plagiarism is the case when two different researchers from two different countries submitted a paper together [4]. Unfortunately the first author, who was not English speaking, copied many sentences from a previous paper [5] onto the first draft and sent it to the English-speaking author who did not notice the identical sentences. However the authors of the original paper [5] sent a letter to the editor of the journal asking the two authors of the manuscript [6] to explain the nature of apparent plagiarism of their manuscript [7]. As Dr. Steve Shafer says: "You will be caught" [8].

Another form of concern can be seen from James C. Eisenach's (Editor in Chief for Anesthesiology) letter [9]. In it he mentions that the same authors submit similar, but not identical, database studies to two different journals. Both got published [10, 11]. Eisenach did not suspect that the data presented in the two papers were fraudulent and that both contributed to patient care. Therefore he did not ask for a retraction. However he states that it is imperative that authors cite "in press" or "published" when submitting their papers to a journal. Failing to do that may be considered duplicitous behavior and may result in a retraction [12–14].

If you are involved with database research, you are advised to read the article by Nafiu and Tremper [15]. In the article, they bring to the attention of the editors the fact that there were considerable overlaps of their two articles which were published in two different journals [16, 17]. Naifiu and Tremper call their paper "Accusation of Salami publication: The new bane of large database investigations? Young investigators beware!" Salami publication is defined as "intentional publication in any form of an article that overlaps substantially with one previously published by the same or different authors" [15]. You may also want to read the editorial by Dr. Steven Shafer [2] about the different forms of plagiarism. They are for your information (1) plagiarism for scientific English, (2) intellectual theft, (3) intellectual sloth, (4) technical plagiarism, and (5) self-plagiarism.

Worse still are publications in which authors describe studies they did not perform. This is fraud and highlighted in an editorial by Eldawlatly and Shafer in 2012 [18]. In it they mention two doctors, Jaydev Dave and Sandip Vaghela, who claim to have performed a study they did not do [19]. They used the same data that had been reported by others [20]. This case and others is serious academic misconduct.

You may think that this does not happen, unfortunately it does. In 2009, Scott Reuben had over 20 research papers retracted [21, 22]. The manuscripts dealt with the use of perioperative nonsteroidal anti-inflammatory drugs. Both results and conclusions were found to be fraudulent. Dr. Joachim Boldt had over 90 papers retracted in 2011 because of no IRB approval [23]. Dr. Yoshitaka Fujii, who was an international expert of postoperative nausea and vomiting, was found to have falsified data in 172 out of 212 papers published between 1993 and 2011 [24] (see Case 58).

So what do you do if you are suspicious of any misdoings?

1. As a reviewer

    You must contact the handling editor and ask him to get the author's institution to start an investigation. You can start with interviewing possible coworkers who were not included on this paper. This may reveal interesting information. Furthermore you can request a copy of the IRB approval for the study. Some journals now require you to produce a copy of the IRB approval when you submit your manuscript.

2. As a coworker

    If you observe what you believe could be misconduct, then you must report it. How you report it and to whom will vary from institution to institution. The institution response to misconduct will be very different from different institutions.

    Other fraudulent activities include attempted duplicate publication, not disclosing conflict of interest correctly, and, as mentioned, attempts at plagiarism.

Lesson

Fraudulent activity will be discovered. The important values as a researcher are that you should be honest, efficient, accurate, and objective. The latter means making the facts speak for themselves and avoid showing any bias.

Today's software can detect plagiarism and academic misconducts.

If you need to reference something verbatim, then always cite your references.

References

1. Shafer SL. Plagiarism and proper English writing: the dilemma (letter). Anesth Analg. 2011;113:664.
2. Shafer SL. You will be caught. Anesth Analg. 2011;112:491–3.
3. Mazoit JX. Plagiarism and proper English writing: the dilemma (letter). Anesth Analg. 2011;113:664.
4. Kihara S, Yaguchi Y, Inomata S, Watanabe S, Brimacombe JR, Taguchi N, et al. Influence of nitrous oxide on minimal alveolar concentration of sevoflurane for laryngeal mask insertion in children. Anesthesiology. 2003;99:1055–8.
5. Swan HD, Crawford MW, Pua HL, Stephens D, Lerman J. Additive contribution of nitrous oxide to sevoflurane minimum alveolar concentration for tracheal intubation in children. Anesthesiology. 1990;91:667–71.
6. Lerman J, Crawford MW. Two manuscripts, too similar. Anesthesiology. 2004;101:801.
7. Kihara S, Brimacombe JR. Two manuscripts, too similar. Anesthesiology. 2004;101:801.
8. Shafer SL (2011) You will be caught. Anesth Analg 112:491–493.
9. Eisenach JC. Note of editorial concern. Anesthesiology. 2011;115:463.
10. Naifu OO, Ramachandran SK, Ackwerh R, Tremper KK, Campbell Jr DA, Stanley JC. Factors associated with and consequences of unplanned post-operative intubation in elderly vascular and general surgery patients. Eur J Anaesthesiol. 2011;28:220–4.
11. Ramachandran SK, Nafiu OO, Ghaferi A, Tremper KK, Shanks A, Kheterpal S. Independent predictors and outcomes of unanticipated early postoperative tracheal intubation after nonemergent, noncardiac surgery. Anesthesiology. 2011;115:44–53.
12. Cotter JT, Nielsen KC, Guller U, Steele SM, Klein SM, Greengrass RA, et al. Increased body mass index and ASA physical status 4 are risk factors for block failure in ambulatory surgery: an analysis of 9,342 blocks. Can J Anesth. 2004;51:810–6.
13. Nielsen KC, Guller U, Steele SM, Klein SM, Greengrass RA, Pietrobon R. Influence of obesity on surgical regional anesthesia in the ambulatory setting: an analysis of 9,038 blocks. Anesthesiology. 2005;102:181–7.
14. Nielsen KC, Guller U, Steele SM, Klein SM, Greengrass RA, Pietrobon R. A lesson learnt. Anesthesiology. 2005;1013:442.
15. Nafiu OO, Tremper KK. Accusation of Salami publications: the new bane of large database investigations? Young investigators beware! Eur J Anaesthesisol. 2011;28:545–6.
16. Nafiu OO, Kheterpal S, Morris M, et al. Incidence and risk factors for preincision hypotension in a noncardiac pediatric surgical population. Paediat Anaesth. 2009;19:232–9.
17. Nafiu OO, Maclean S, Blum J, et al. High BMI in children as a risk factor for intraoperative hypotension. Eur J Anaesthesiol. 2010;27:1065–68.
18. Eldawlaty A, Shafer SL. Caveat lector. Anesth Analg. 2012;114:1160–2.
19. Dave J, Vaghela S. A comparison of the sedative, hemodynamic, and respiratory effects of dexmedetomidine and propofol in children undergoing magnetic resonance imaging. Saudi J Anaesth. 2011;5:295–9.
20. Koroglu A, Teksan H, Sagir O, Yucel A, Toprak H, Erosy O. A comparison of the sedative, hemodynamic and respiratory effects of dexmedetomidine and propofol in children undergoing magnetic resonance imaging. Anesth Analgl. 2006;103:63–7.
21. Shafer SL. Retraction. Anesth Analg. 2009;108:1350.
22. Heckman JD. Retraction. J Bone Joint Surg Am. 2009;91:965.
23. Shafer SL. Notice of retraction. Anesth Analg. 2010;111:1567.
24. Fujii Y. Retraction. Int J Gynaecol Obstet. 2013;120(1):109.

Chapter 45
Case 45: Pediatric Research

A fellow in pediatric anesthesiology approaches you with a suggested clinical research study. He is interested in developing a safe sedation/anesthetic management protocol for uncooperative children undergoing magnetic resonance imaging (MRI). He has come across a case report by Rosen and Daume [1] where they described an uncooperative child for an MRI using intravenous dexmedetomidine. The drug is not recommended for use in children. Unfortunately they made a miscalculation, and instead of a bolus, they gave the drug as a continuous infusion which resulted in a tenfold overdose. Your fellow tells you that the child tolerated the overdose and was discharged to home the same day. This fact, the fellow states, must mean that the drug is safe and could potentially be used for sedation/anesthesia in these cases. Furthermore, the case was published by a reputable journal.

What is your response to this request? What are the concerns?

© Springer Science+Business Media New York 2015

J.G. Brock-Utne, *Clinical Research*, DOI 10.1007/978-1-4939-2516-2_45

Answer/Solution

There are several concerns. In no particular order:

1. Dexmedetomidine was used as an off-label drug in this child. It was also used in an excessive amount. But as Tobin, Shafer, and Davis wonder [2]: "whether it is appropriate to publish an off-label use of a drug, particularly when it is further compromised by an inadvertent tenfold overdose." I would think that the authors were brave to publish the result of their misadventure and the editor was correct in publishing it, as it serves as an important data point [2].
2. It is a sad fact that nearly 85 % of drugs in the Physicians' Desk Reference do not have labeled indications for children [2]. However, off-labeled drugs are often prescribed to children with dose adjustments based mainly on weight. Unfortunately side effects in children when using these drugs are often not predicted because of differences in pharmacokinetics and pharmacodynamics [3].
3. An investigational use of the drug (IND) must be sought. This is obviously imperative for unapproved new drugs. But the FDA may also require an IND when an approved drug is to be used off-label. The FDA Web site should be helpful to researchers to determine if their proposed study will require FDA review (http://www.fda.gov/cder/guidance/phase1.pdf). As a guideline, if you are seeking to change the drug label with your study, like in this case, then an IND application is required. The FDA most likely will insist that the pharmaceutical companies should perform all clinical research under an IND.

If you are uncertain if an IND application is need, you should contact the FDA prior to starting a study.

The advantages of an IND application are many. The FDA can tell you if a trial like the one you are proposing has failed before (not published) and that the drug has caused organ toxicity in an animal model dealing with growth and development. They can also advise you on how to safely monitor patients and what to look out for. An FDA review, if an IND is needed, should take no more than 30 days [4].

Discussion

Fortunately there are many safeguards to protect children who participate in clinical research. Most commonly these studies are started and supported by the pharmaceutical industry. Their responsibility is simple. They must disclose all know risks associated with the drug so that the parents/guardians can make an educated decision on whether to allow the child to participate in the study.

It is not recommended to do a trial that requires an IND without an FDA approval. If you do and the FDA finds out, then the FDA will perform an inspection of the research site to ascertain any risks to the subjects. The magnitude of the risk to research subjects will be incorporated in the assessment, and there may be legal actions brought against you and the institution. Also remember that even a dietary supplement or a chemical not obtained from a pharmacy requires an IND.

It is well know that pharmacokinetics (PK) and pharmacodynamics (PD) and safety studies are needed to determine the correct dose of drugs [5]. There are several problems attempting to determine PK/PD in children. The amount of blood draws is prohibited in both neonates and infants. The other problem is that these studies should also be conducted in healthy children, not only the ones who may benefit from the drug [6]. Sick children may have underlying renal and hepatic disease, and concurrent treatment may affect drugs kinetics or dose response. Also adult body metabolism and composition may preclude direct translation of dosage guidelines to children [7].

To increase the number of pediatric clinical trials, the US Congress (1997) passed the Food and Drug Administration Modernization Act (FDAMA). This provided incentives in the form of a 6-month extension of patent or marketing exclusivity for conducting pediatric clinical trials for drugs already approved for use in adults. It is debatable if this has been helpful.

In a non-industry-sponsored pediatric study [8], we saw firsthand the lack of cooperation and/or sheer obstruction by a pharmaceutical company, IRB, and one editor to whom we sent our paper. Finally it got accepted by Editor in Chief Ted Sumner in Pediatric Anesthesia. Well-designed and executed clinical trials in children are of paramount importance, so that this group of patients can be given drugs safely.

Lesson

Drug research in pediatrics is complex. An IND may be needed. Be mindful of any suggestions from the FDA.

References

1. Rosen DA, Daume JT. Short duration high dose dexmedetomidine in a pediatric patient during procedural sedation. Anesth Analg. 2006;103:68–9.
2. Tobin JR, Shafer SL, Davis PJ. Pediatric research and scholarship: another Gordian knot? Anesth Analg. 2006;103:43–8.
3. Anderson BJ, Hansen TG. Getting the best from pediatric pharmacokinetic data. Paediatr Anaesth. 2004;14:713–5.
4. Schultheis LW, Mathis LL, Roca RAQ, Simone AF, Hertz SH, Rappaport BA. Pediatric drug development in anesthesiology: an FDA perspective. Anesth Analg. 2006;103:49–51.
5. Schreiner MS, Greeley WJ. Pediatric clinical trials: shall we take a lead? Anesth Analg. 2002;94:1–3.
6. Wilson JT, Kearns GL, Murphy D, Yaffe SJ. Paediatric labeling requirements: implications for further studies. Clin Pharmacokinet. 1994;26:308–25.
7. Bokesch PM. (letter) Untying the Gordian knot. Anesth Analg. 2006;103:249.
8. Lammers CR, Rosner JL, Crockett DE, Chhokra R, Brock-Utne JG. Oral midazolam with an antacid may increase the speed of onset of sedation in children prior to general anaesthesia. Paediatr Anaesthesia. 2002;12:1–4.

Chapter 46
Case 46: Your Paper Is Rejected. What to Do

Your manuscript is rejected. You are devastated, as this is, as far as you can ascertain, the largest English language randomized study done on this topic. The journal, to which you submitted your work, has published previous work on this topic. You feel that your manuscript adds new information to the literature. Although the study shows no difference between the groups, the results are economically important, as one group's treatment is cheaper than the other and equally as effective.

What would you do? Give up, find another journal, or resubmit to the journal that rejected it?

© Springer Science+Business Media New York 2015
J.G. Brock-Utne, *Clinical Research*, DOI 10.1007/978-1-4939-2516-2_46

Answer/Solution

I rarely resubmit a paper to the same journal that has rejected it. But in this case based on what is stated on the previous page, I would write a letter something like this:

Dear Editor,

It is with great regret that we note your rejection of our paper. We appreciate you and your reviewer's hard work and time dedicated to reviewing our submission. The reason for your rejection was that our paper did not get sufficient priority. We respectfully ask that you look at it again. The reasons are several. This is, as far as we can ascertain, the largest English language randomized study done on this topic. We feel it adds new information to the literature, and since your journal has published on this topic, your journal would be an ideal choice. Although the study showed no difference between the groups, the result is economically important, as one group's treatment is cheaper than the other and both are equally effective. Please note that the study is adequately powered.

In light of this, we urge you to review our submission again.

Yours sincerely

Lesson

If you feel strongly that the paper belongs in the journal that rejected it, then resubmit it to the same journal. Always include a cover letter explaining why you want the editor to reconsider. If it still gets rejected, then submit elsewhere.

Chapter 47
Case 47: You Disagree with a Conclusion of a Published Article

You have read an original article published in a respected journal [1]. You and your colleagues find the title misleading as it infers that only one parameter (low tidal volumes) can improve patient outcome following intermittent positive pressure ventilation (IPPV).

You decide to write a letter to the editor which is summarized below:

"In the study [1], in ventilated ICU patients, there were two interventional groups. Group 1 used only high tidal volumes during intermittent positive pressure ventilation (IPPV), while group 2 used lower tidal volume but also included positive end-expiratory pressure (PEEP) and a lung recruitment maneuver (periodic hyper-inflation of the lungs) every 30 min. Each of these three interventions (low tidal volume, PEEP, and periodic hyperinflation) in group 2 may have independently influenced the outcome of this study. The relative importance of each of these parameters in the minimization of postoperative pulmonary complications was not tested in this study and remains a topic of controversy.

We bring this to your readership's attention as we suspect some may take away the message that it is only low tidal volumes that affects the outcome of the study. They must not forget to include PEEP and periodic recruitment in the multifactor lung protective ventilation strategy."

Your letter (above) was rejected by the editor of the journal and no comment was given.

What will you do? Give up?

© Springer Science+Business Media New York 2015
J.G. Brock-Utne, *Clinical Research*, DOI 10.1007/978-1-4939-2516-2_47

Answer/Solution

You should submit your letter to another journal like one that deals with anesthesia and ICU. In the letter, you should state that the paper provides a potentially misguided interpretation.

Discussion

The reason you want to inform your anesthesia colleagues is that hospital committees and other physicians may want to change ICU ventilator practice based on this paper. By informing your colleagues and committee members, you are providing knowledge of the paper and its shortcomings.

In another example [2], the editor refused a letter to the correspondence section of the journal from clinicians who were concerned about the conclusion of the paper [2]. These physicians managed to get their concerns published in an anesthesia journal [3]. In the original article [2], the implication was that anesthetic techniques (regional or general) were a risk factor for stroke in *ALL* surgical patients. But the article [2] only looked at patients who had undergone from cardiac, vascular, and maxillofacial surgery cases. They had therefore not considered all surgical cases.

Lesson

Always consider writing to the editor about a published paper when you feel the conclusions may misguide clinicians or hospital administrators.

References

1. Futier E, Constantin J-M, Paugam-Burtz C, Pascal J, Eurin M, Neuschwander A, Marret E, Beaussier M, Gutton C, Lefrant J-Y, Allaouchiche B, Verzilli D, Leone M, De Jong A, Bazin J-E, Pereira B, Jaber S. (Improve study group). A trial of intraoperative low-tidal-volume ventilation in abdominal surgery. NEMJ. 2013;369:428–37.
2. Salem M. Perioperative stroke. NEMJ. 2007;356:706–13.
3. Dunstan C, Jerwood C. Perioperative stroke: implications of anesthetic technique. Anaesthesia. 2007;62:853.

Chapter 48
Case 48: Is This a Good Study?

You are an attending physician in a large university hospital. An ENT resident suggests the following clinical study: a comparison of a new oral hypotensive agent about which you know nothing to a placebo. The drug is to be given 48 h prior to surgery. The study is to be prospective, double blinded, and randomized. The objective is to improve surgical conditions as assessed by a blinded surgeon. If published, the resident hopes to add to the control hypotension/bleeding literature. He plans to use a Mann–Whitney U test.

Have you any concerns about this study as described above? If so, what?

© Springer Science+Business Media New York 2015
J.G. Brock-Utne, *Clinical Research*, DOI 10.1007/978-1-4939-2516-2_48

Answer/Solution

There are several concerns with this study. In no particular order, they are:

1. It is nearly always better to compare a new drug or treatment modality to an active control group.
2. What class is the new drug being investigated? A drug given 48 h preoperatively may not be the safest and most convenient choice. Prolonged or even dangerous intraoperative hypotension may result.
3. Has the drug ever been studied in this setting? If so, what were the results? What does the packet insert say?
4. A Friedman's test for nonparametric data may prove to be more appropriate.
5. It is imperative that the anesthetic drugs and ventilator settings including tidal volume and PEEP are the same for each group.
6. It is important that all patients be placed in the same position, for example, reverse Trendelenburg.
7. Has the new drug any effect on the bioavailability of anesthetic drugs, antibiotics, etc.?
8. Is the only study looking at one oral dose or several?
9. What are the rescue drugs to be used in both groups should the blood pressure be too low or two high?

Lesson

Always investigate and discuss in detail any proposed clinical research study. This will save you a lot of time and frustration as often a badly conceived study will not be published.

Chapter 49
Case 49: Meta-analysis of Randomized Controlled Trials

You are a new faculty member at a university hospital. There is an expectation that you will do research. A senior member of the department approaches you with a potential study. He wants you to be the principal investigator. The study involves examining/reviewing several meta-analysis randomized controlled trials. In this case, the object is to compare a single-shot femoral nerve blockade (SSFNB) to continuous femoral nerve block (CFNB) for analgesia after a total knee arthroplasty. You state that you will learn more about meta-analysis, review all the articles on the subject, and then get back to him in a week. You tell him that you are delighted and grateful for the offer.

You find out that a meta-analysis can increase statistical power by pooling and analyzing results from several comparable studies. But the results and conclusions of any single study are as good as the data analyzed. If the results are based on biased and confounding data, then the validity of the meta-analysis conclusions will be suspect.

After you have reviewed the various individual studies which are to be included in the meta-analysis, supplied by your colleague, you find only two comparable studies with a total of 69 patients. Interestingly both these two studies have come to two totally different conclusions.

What will you do? Decline or accept the offer?

If you accept, will you include in your meta-analysis study those studies that do not come from a randomized comparison, so as to increase the numbers?

© Springer Science+Business Media New York 2015
J.G. Brock-Utne, *Clinical Research*, DOI 10.1007/978-1-4939-2516-2_49

Answer/Solution

1. I would decline the offer.
2. Never include in your meta-analysis study those studies that do not come from a randomized comparison (for discussion, see below).

Discussion

Paul et al. [1] published a meta-analysis of the above problem from 23 randomized controlled trials, but only two trials (n-69) were a direct comparison of SSFNB to CFNB [2, 3]. It is worthwhile reading the criticism of their article by Barrington et al. [3]. In summary Barrington et al. make the following concerns about the article by Paul et al. [1]:

1. There were only two studies that had a direct comparison [3, 4].
2. In these two studies [3, 4], different local anesthetics (bupivacaine and ropivacaine) were used, although Paul et al. felt that this was not really important since a study [5] had shown no difference in the block effectiveness. The surgery was also noted to be different.
3. Inclusion of published non-randomized studies.
4. The conclusion by Paul et al. was that: "these studies do not demonstrate further improvement with continuous femoral nerve block, compared with single-shot femoral nerve block." Barrington et al. stated that the only conclusion of Paul's study [1] could have was: "that there is conflicting evidence and more studies are required to determine which techniques are most appropriate for femoral nerve blockade for total knee arthoplasty."

The quality of randomized controlled trials (RCT) in major anesthesiology journals has been studied [6]. Significant improvement in the reporting and conduct of RCT is required. Special attention should focus on randomization methodology, the blinding of investigators, and the size of the sample studied. They [6] also recommend adopting guidelines for the improvement of the quality of randomized controlled trials.

One problem that is seen in meta-analysis results is that the analyses were conducted over several years, sometimes 20 years. Obviously medical treatments, monitoring, etc. have changed over such a long time span, making any comparison difficult. An example of the latter is the 2009 article by Wilder et al. [7] who reported their finding of a retrospective cohort study of anesthetic exposure and learning disabilities between 1976 and 1982. They reported that patients younger than 4 years old who had two or more exposures to general anesthesia had a greater proportion of learning disabilities compared with children who had one or no exposure to general anesthesia. This article indicated a detrimental effect of general anesthesia on the developing brain. They concluded that anesthesia in infancy is linked to later learning disabilities. However, the authors overlooked the fact that the majority of the children in their study were anesthetized before the routine use of pulse oximetry. Pulse oximetry was developed in the 1970s and only became commonly used at the end of the 1980s [8, 9]. There is no doubt that the use of pulse oximetry produced a great reduction in the incidence of undetected hypoxia and resultant injury [10]. Since the children in Wilder et al. study received general anesthesia from 1976 to 1982, it is therefore possible that the increased incidence of learning difficulties might have resulted in part from an undetected and therefore not documented hypoxia. This article by Wilder et al. sparked a lot of criticism [9, 11–13] like not be able to adjust for comorbidity like children with cerebral palsy, history of meningitis, etc. invalidates any conclusion from the study [11]

Another concern is that meta-analysis often does not detail any conflict of interest, like industry funding or author-industry financial ties for each individual study. This information is important to include in the meta-analysis study so that the reader can appraise the meta-analyses study conclusion.

Lesson

If you are doing a meta-analysis study, then you need to study only head-to-head comparisons. If you don't, then you may make inappropriate conclusions.

Don't forget to give details of any conflict of interest in all the studies included in the meta-analysis.

References

1. Paul JE, Arya A, Hurlburt L, Cheng J, Thabane L, Tidy A, Murthy Y. Femoral nerve block improves analgesia outcomes after total knee arthroplasty. A meta-analysis of randomized controlled trials. Anesthesiology. 2010;113:1014–5.
2. Hirst GC, Lang SA, Dust WN, Cassidy JD, Yip RW. Femoral nerve block: single injection versus continuous infusion for total knee arthroplasty. Region Anesth. 1996;21:292–7.
3. Salinas FV, Liu SS, Mulroy MF. The effect of single-injection femoral nerve block versus continuous femoral nerve block after total knee arthroplasty on hospital length of stay and long-term functional recovery within an established clinical pathway. Anesth Analg. 2006;102:1234–9.
4. Barrington MJ, Olive DJ, Kluger R. Inappropriate conclusion from meta-analysis of randomized controlled trials. Anesth Analg. 2011;114:1494–5.
5. Wulf H, Lowe J, Gnutzmann KH, Steinfeldt T. Femoral nerve block with ropivacaine or bupivacaine in day case anterior crucial ligament reconstructions. Acta Anaesth Scand. 2010;54:414–20.
6. Greenfield MLVH, Rosenberg AL, O'Reilly M, Shanks AM, Sliwinski MJ, Nauss MD. The quality of randomized controlled trials in major anesthesiology journals. Anesth Analg. 2005;100:159–64.
7. Wilder RT, Flick RP, Sprung J, Katusic SK, Barbaresi WJ, Mickelson C, Gleich SJ, Schroeder DR, Weaver AL, Warner DO. Early exposure to anesthesia and learning disabilities in a population-based birth cohort. Anesthesiology. 2009;110:796–804.

8. Severinghaus JW, Honda Y. History of blood gas analysis. VII: Pulse oximetry. J Clin Monit. 1987;3:135–8.
9. Mitchell JA. Learning disabilities may be related to undetected hypoxia (letter). Anesthesiology. 2009;111:1379.
10. Eichhorn JH. Prevention of intraoperative anesthesia accidents and related severe injury through safety monitoring. Anesthesiology. 1989;70:572–7.
11. Sturen Arul G, Thies K-C. The elephant in the room. Anesthesiology. 2009;111:1380.
12. Cote CJ. Learning disabilities and repeated anesthetics: drugs or airway management issues? Anesthesiology. 2009;111:1379–80.
13. Tolpin DA, Collard CD. If the odds are a million to one against something occurring, chances are 50–50 it will. Anesthesiology. 2009;111:1380–1.

Chapter 50
Case 50: Is the Title of a Paper or Grant Important?

You are writing a case report. It deals with an unusual capnograph tracing that developed during a general anesthetic in an otherwise healthy adult. The trace is triphasic with an initial lower plateau, followed by a higher plateau (hump) and then followed by a lower plateau. This has not been described before. Your medical student tells you it looks like a dromedary.

You are considering calling the paper "An unusual capnograph tracing" but dismiss it as you think it sounds too boring.

What would be your suggestion in this example?

What are your ideas for making the title more interesting?

© Springer Science+Business Media New York 2015
J.G. Brock-Utne, *Clinical Research*, DOI 10.1007/978-1-4939-2516-2_50

Answer/Solution

"The Dromedary sign – an unusual capnograph tracing" [1]

Discussion

The title of both a manuscript and a grant application are more important than many researchers realize. It should be concise, but should describe the content of your manuscript/application. The title should stand out from others. It should encourage the reviewers and eventually the reader to read your paper. Try and make it unique and relevant like: "Failure to ventilate with the Drager Apollo Anesthesia Work Station" [2] or: "A poor correlation exists between oscillometric and radial arterial blood pressure as measured by the Phillips MP70 monitor " [3].

It can be useful to pose a question in your title, for example, "Myocardial ischemia after electroconvulsive therapy (ECT): are cardiac troponin levels useful?" [4] or "Is there an optimum location to measure noninvasive blood pressure in morbidly obese patients?" [5] or "Heat moisture exchange devices. Are they doing what they are supposed to do?"[6].

Attempt to have a title with no more than 80–100 characters. Note that some granting agencies or journals may have specific requirements.

If you are applying for a grant, the title should inform the reviewers of the essence of the project. For instance, you could pose a question which indicates what you want to do or you could point to the possible outcome of the research in your title.

Also chose the words carefully in the title so they can be picked up by search engines [7].

Lesson

Make sure that the title is both relevant and original and differs substantially from other grants or papers which have been submitted or published on the subject. The title can be the key to success in obtaining a grant or having your paper accepted.

References

1. Jaffe RA, Talavera JA, Hah JM, Brock-Utne JG. The dromedary sign – an unusual capnograph tracing. Anesthesiology. 2008;109:149–50.
2. Hilton G, Moll V, Zumaran AA, Jaffe RA, Brock-Utne JG. Failure to ventilate with the Drager Apollo Anesthesia workstation. Anesthesiology. 2011;114:1138–242.

3. Mireles SA, Jaffe RA, Drover D, Brock-Utne JG. A poor correlation exists between oscillometric and radial arterial blood pressure as measured by the Phillips MP70 monitor. J Clin Invest. 2009;23:169–74.
4. Hennessey EK, Solvason HB, Brock-Utne JG Myocardial ischemia after ECT: are cardiac troponin levels useful? 2014 (in press).
5. Anast N, Olejniczak M, Brock-Utne JG, Ingrande J, Jaffe JA, Lemmens HJM. Is there an optimum location to measure non-invasive blood pressure in morbidly obese patients? Presented at American Society Annual meeting, 19–23 October 2012, Washington DC.
6. Lemmens HJM, Brock-Utne JG. Heat and moisture exchange devices. Are they doing what they are supposed to do? Anesth Analg. 2004;98:382–5.
7. Davison AJ, Carlin JB. What a reviewer wants (A review article). Pediatr Anesth. 2008;18:1149–56.

Chapter 51
Case 51: Sampling and Subjects

You are writing a research manuscript. The paper reports on the use of two different therapeutic management techniques in patients with insulin-dependent diabetes mellitus.

You describe the patient population as such: "eighty-five patients from the hospital diabetes mellitus clinic were included in the study."

Is this an acceptable statement? What is missing?

© Springer Science+Business Media New York 2015
J.G. Brock-Utne, *Clinical Research*, DOI 10.1007/978-1-4939-2516-2_51

Answer/Solution

No, this is not an acceptable statement.

Discussion

You must also tell the reader from where the patients got referred. A better wording would be:

"Patients were identified in a hospital mellitus clinic at a university center. 65 % were referred from the hospital emergency room, 25 % from other hospital clinics and 10 % from physicians in the nearby district."

The description of your selection sampling is important. You should tell where the sampling took place, over what period of time, who was eligible to participate, how many were asked to participate, how many entered the trial, and how many completed the trial.

Stating 85 patients does not tell the reader how many were actually eligible, how many started, and how many completed the trial. The sentence should be something like this: 130 patients were eligible, 22 patient refused to participate, 31 did not fulfill the practical study criteria, and 7 patients did not complete the study, leaving 70 patients, who were randomly assigned to two groups. In these cases, it is often advisable to make a flow diagram over the breakdown of patients and also of how they fared after they were randomized.

As concerns the randomization, it is imperative to say something like this: "The patients were randomly assigned by a nurse coordinator, who opened a sealed envelope with a number which had been previously generated by a random number table. The number was then assigned to the patient". The two groups' characteristics, as well as those that did not complete the study, should be shown in a Table. There were no statistically significant differences in any single characteristic. There was a trend (but not significant) that more men than women decided not to participate.

It is also important to state when the study started and ended, for example, from November 30, 2013, to December 1, 2014).

Mention must also be made of sample size and statistical power. An example would be: Assuming a control group response of 20 % and using a two-sided type I error=0.05 and type II error=0.20 (power=0.8), sample size calculations indicate that 35 subjects in each group would provide an 80 % power for an absolute difference of 15 %.

Lesson

It is important to use the correct method terminology if you want your work to be fully understood by the reader and accepted for publication.

Chapter 52
Case 52: What Not to Do If You Are a Mentor

You have been appointed as a Departmental Mentor and Facilitator of Resident's and Fellow's Research in a medical department. You are excited about the job.

A resident has been given research time and money for a specific laboratory project to develop a new patient cooling device. She now wants to change the project. This is because recent published work indicates that this line of research has no longer any merit. The resident has used some of the previously allocated research fund ($1,500 out of total $8,000). She wants to use the remaining funds for her new research project which is the development of a new blood warming device. She also wants to get an additional $2,000.00 in support and wonders if these requests to alter direction and to obtain extra funding can be expedited, as she is starting her allocated 8-week laboratory research in 1 week.

Prior to sending this request to the research committee, you must get detailed information in writing about how the funds to date have been spent, why the resident wants to change direction, and how much is needed for the new project. Finally she should explain if her new warming device may lead to a medical product and if so who will own the patent?

What else must you do?

© Springer Science+Business Media New York 2015
J.G. Brock-Utne, *Clinical Research*, DOI 10.1007/978-1-4939-2516-2_52

Answer/Solution

You must deal with this as soon as possible since the resident starts her allocated research time in 1 week.

Discussion

If you take on a role as a Departmental Mentor and Facilitator of Resident's and Fellow's Research, then it is imperative to consider that their research is just as important as yours. You must encourage them in their endeavors and be available 24/7 to deal with their problems/concerns in a timely and efficient manner. If you do that, then your support should help them remain enthusiastic and interested in their research, even when they hit difficult patches. If you are not available for advice, the residents/fellows can easily become disheartened and uninterested in doing further research.

I have seen a case where the mentor sent the resident's application to the research committee for a change of both direction and funding. The mentor, on behalf of the resident, asked for a quick decision. Within 2 days, the committee approved the application, but the mentor was too busy to inform the resident. There was a delay of over 3 weeks, leaving only 6 out of the 8 weeks to finish the project. It was only by chance that the resident asked a member of the research committee for the status of her request and was told that the application had been approved and that their decision had been conveyed to the mentor. On further investigation, it turned out that the mentor had been too focused on his own research and family matters to have the time to inform the resident. In this case, the mentor should have asked another faculty member, preferably from the research committee, to speak/write to the resident and outline the research committee's recommendation and requirements. It is no shame to delegate work. There will always come a time when one is too busy to carry out all ones duties.

To be a good mentor, you need to be enthusiastic about the mentee's research. You need to listen carefully to their concerns and ideas and be supportive at all time. For the mentees and at time also the mentor to fully understand the field of research, it is a good idea for the mentee to write a review article on their chosen topic. A lot of questions will be generated from this review. As a mentor, you should inspire your mentee and be easily approachable and not cause fear and trepidations. Always instill in the mentee to look out for any possible conflict of interest.

Lesson

It is not easy to be a good mentor, but you should always remember that the mentee's research and deadlines are as important as your own.

As a mentor, you should fully understand the topic/question the mentee is researching; failure to do that is a gross disservice to the mentee.

Chapter 53
Case 53: Be Aware

You are an associate professor in surgery at a famous university medical center. You get a phone call from a colleague, who is also an associate professor in surgery, at another university medical center. He tells you that he is including you as an author on a paper he is about to submit. He says he is doing this in appreciation of all the preliminary discussions you had with him before he started the study.

You are a bit taken aback, as you feel that your small contribution does not warrant authorship. You tell him not to include you, but he is very insistent that he wants to do so.

What would you do now?

© Springer Science+Business Media New York 2015

J.G. Brock-Utne, *Clinical Research*, DOI 10.1007/978-1-4939-2516-2_53

Answer/Solution

Ask him to send you the final version of the manuscript and then you will decide if you want to be included as an author.

Discussion

The case of Dr. Yoshitaka Fujii is a case in point. Dr. Fujii, as mentioned (Case 44), had published over 170 papers on nausea and vomiting postoperatively. He had become an international expert in this field. A reviewer of his latest manuscript got very suspicious, as all of Dr. Fujii's antiemetic drug results had almost identical side effects. The reviewer got a statistician to go over the stats [1]. He wanted him to evaluate whether the published distributions of various variables were consistent with the distributions what could be expected to result from random chance. The statistician concluded that the data sets were "extremely unlikely to have arisen by chance." He noted that many of the distributions had "likelihoods that were infinitesimally small" about 1 in 150 million.

This led to an investigation by an ethical committee who reported that of the 249 papers credited to Dr. Fujii, 172 papers contained falsified data. Dr. Fujii later retracted the paper [2–4].

What was also concerning was that Dr. Fujii included doctors from other institutions to make his paper look like it was a multicenter study. To make matters even worse, many of the authors on his papers were not aware that they had been included as coworkers!

Lesson

When someone offers you an authorship, you must peruse and agree with the final version of the paper before it is sent to a journal. If you feel unsure about the results and if your involvement has been very little, then turn down the offer. Document your refusal in an email; preferably also inform the editor of the journal to which it is being submitted.

References

1. Carlisle JB. An analysis of 168 randomized controlled trials to test data integrity. Anesthesia. 2012;67:521–37.
2. Fujii Y. Retraction. Int J Gynaecol Obstet. 2013;120(1):109.
3. Shafer SL. Notice of retraction. Anesth Analg. 2012;115:982.
4. Shafer SL. Notice of retraction. Anesth Analg. 2010;111:1567.

Chapter 54
Case 54: A Statistical Impasse

We submitted a paper dealing with the impact of positive end expiratory pressure (PEEP) (0.5–10 cm H_2O) on the right internal jugular vein (RIJV) cross-sectional area (CSA) in obese patients. Other studies have looked at this question but we decided to examine both the impact of RIJA CSA as well as the cardiovascular tolerance to the increased PEEP. Each patient acted as his/her own control. This question had not been addressed before. We found an increase in CSA associated with the increased PEEP, but there was a 25 % incidence of patient cardiovascular intolerance to the increased PEEP. Our statistical analysis was with a two paired Student's *t*-test.

The paper was provisionally accepted, but one reviewer out of three wanted us to do a linear regression using PEEP on the *x*-axis and percentage change on the *y*-axis. We went to the university statistic department who told us that: "Linear regression is not the ideal test to do in this case. In actual fact, performing the two paired Student's *t*-test on this data is a textbook example of when this test should be used."

Now what will you do?

© Springer Science+Business Media New York 2015
J.G. Brock-Utne, *Clinical Research*, DOI 10.1007/978-1-4939-2516-2_54

Answer/Solution

Do the linear regression and resubmit with both statistical methods.

Discussion

The arguments for the *t*-test over the linear regression are (a) there is no reason to suspect a linear relationship between PEEP and CSA, (b) a linear relationship is not required to show a clinically significant effect, and (c) we have no assumption or interest in a dose-dependent effect and so a linear regression is unnecessary.

We resubmitted the paper, including both tests in the methods. Interestingly both tests yielded similar results. We asked the editor if we could publish only the Student *t*-test results. The paper was then returned to us. We were asked more questions regarding the statistics, and the corresponding editor insisted that we include the results of both statistical tests in our submission. We answered the questions and reluctantly agreed to have both statistical test published. After this resubmission, we got even more questions from the one reviewer who dealt with the statistics. At that point, we contacted the editor in chief to get a clarification if the journal wanted to publish our paper. If not, we would then seek publication elsewhere. The editor told us to resubmit which we did. The paper is now in press.

Lesson

It can be arduous to get papers published today. Please remember always to be courteous in your dealings with the editor and the reviewers. If, for whatever reason, you decide not to pursue publication in a journal that has provisionally accepted your work, then you must inform the editor and reviewers of your decision to withdraw your paper. This should be in the form of a written withdrawal.

Chapter 55
Case 55: A Bad Outcome

You are doing a clinical study on a new intravenous (IV) antiemetic which has been promoted to reduce/prevent postoperative nausea and vomiting. The drug is to be given about 90 min before the end of the surgery.

One study patient is a 74-year-old male ASA 2 coming for an open radical prostatectomy. The patient's previous anesthetics had been uneventful and he has no allergies. His past history is significant for hypertension and coronary artery disease. The surgeon is informed of the study and has no objection to the patient's participation. The patient consented to the study in the preoperative area and is taken back to the operating room. After monitors are placed, the patient is given a routine general anesthetic and the surgery starts. As is customary, this surgeon plays his favorite music very loudly. The patient's vital signs are stable at the time the study drug is given IV. The blood loss has been about 500 mL. Two to four minutes after the antiemetic is given, the blood pressure falls precipitously and the heart rate increases to over 140 bpm. Through the noise of the music, you ask the surgeon if there is any excess blood loss. The reply is: "Average and nothing to be concerned about." You suspect, the patient has had an allergic reaction to the antiemetic and treat him with epinephrine, etc. However, despite all resuscitation attempts, the patient dies on the operating room table.

You are devastated. If this was not an allergic reaction, what could it have been?

© Springer Science+Business Media New York 2015

J.G. Brock-Utne, *Clinical Research*, DOI 10.1007/978-1-4939-2516-2_55

Answer/Solution

This happened to a friend of mine. He was convinced the cardiovascular collapse was due to an allergic reaction caused by the antiemetic drug, since the surgeon had informed him that the blood loss was "average and nothing to be concerned about." The blood loss could not be verified because firstly the suction could not be heard due to the music and secondly the blood was sucked into a wall suction, which could not be seen. Hence, my friend was unable to detect the excessive blood loss, which was later discovered to be over 3 L.

In this case, it was easy to presume that the cause of the hypotension was related to the study drug.

Lesson

1. In situations like this think: "Commonest things are the commonest" (as my old Professor of Surgery, Jack Henry, Trinity College, Dublin, always said).
2. Blood loss in these operations will always be the commonest cause of hypotension and tachycardia.
3. Never jump to conclusions. Always check your facts. In this case, if you had discovered the blood loss and given blood, the patient would probably have survived.
4. Turn off the OR music when a patient's vital signs becomes unstable.
5. Be wary if the wall suctions do not have a visual collection system. Fortunately these are no longer recommended. But that does not mean they don't exist.

Chapter 56
Case 56: A Case Report

From time to time you will, in your clinical practice, come across an interesting/unusual case. If you feel it is of significant clinical importance, you may want to have your case report published so as to share your experience with others. An example of such a case is the following which happened to us.

We cancelled a general anesthetic for a surgical procedure on the day of surgery. The case was a 35-year-old patient (65 kg, 5′9) with a preoperative resting heart rate of 110 in sinus rhythm. Since there was no clinical reason for having an elevated heart rate (no fever, a normal physical exam, no pain, and a normal TSH), we sent an urgent urine toxicology screen to the laboratory. Thirty minutes later, the results came back positive for amphetamines. When the patient was questioned again about possible illicit drug use, he adamantly denied ever using any.

The patient was furious that his surgery was cancelled, even though he was told that if he had had a general anesthetic with such a large amount of amphetamines present, it could have been fatal. The patient was told by the surgeon that he would not operate until he had three consecutive negative urine samples for illicit drugs. The patient departed and never returned.

We wanted to submit this as a case report. The object was to warn the anesthesia community to be acutely aware of an unexplained preoperative tachycardia in an otherwise healthy patient. However, there was a problem. Since 2010, the patient must give informed consent for the case to be published in which he or she is featured, even though all personal identifiers would be removed in the report. The consent from the patient must be stated at the end of the introduction section.

I knew that the above patient would not give his informed consent and I did not even consider asking him.

Left with this dilemma, what would you do to try and get this case report published?

© Springer Science+Business Media New York 2015   149
J.G. Brock-Utne, *Clinical Research*, DOI 10.1007/978-1-4939-2516-2_56

Answer/Solution

I contacted the university IRB and asked for their policy in this regard.

Discussion

Our IRB did not consider the case report to constitute research (other IRBs may require a review by the IRB). We submitted our case with this sentence at the end of the introduction. However, the editor of the journal refused to review our submission, stating that all case reports must have a written approval from the patient to publish, even though no identifiers were included in the report.

It is important to realize that although all identifiers may be removed from the case report description, the patient may still recognize himself/herself from the unusual nature of the case. Also the names of the authors and place of work are always mentioned.

Other journals may not be so strict. Ideally you should contact either the patient or the patient's legal designee for consent to divulge some of the patient's protected health information. If you are able to obtain consent, all is well. This fact should be stated at the end of the introduction section of your case report.

If you have made reasonable attempts to contact the patient but have been unsuccessful, then you must contact your IRB. If the IRB agrees that you can submit your case for publication, then you must write the following sentence at the end of the Introduction section: "We have made multiple attempts to contact the patient or their legal designee but have been unsuccessful. We have sought approval from our IRB, who gave permission to seek publication of our case report. Furthermore, our IRB determined that an IRB approval was not required."

It is important to realize that your IRB policy *DOES NOT* override the journal's policy to make "reasonable attempts" to obtain permission. The journals will warn you that failure to follow their policy as outlined above will result in delaying the processing of your submission or in denying for it to be sent for peer review. You are advised to review the Guide to Authors prior to sending in your submission.

In a letter to the editor, Hubregtse and Collins [1] tell of an interesting rare complication related to spinal anesthesia. Before they asked for permission from the patient to publish the report, the hospital secretary told the authors not to submit their case report. The secretary had learned that the patient's relatives had expressed their intent to institute legal proceedings against the hospital. Even though no negligence had been suggested, the authors agreed not to publish their report. The hospital maintained: "that the clinical details could leave the hospital a 'disastrous hostage to fortune' in view of the potential magnitude of the claim." It was obviously important in this case not to publish. Hence, obtaining consent from the patient serves as a guide as to what the patient or relatives feel about the "so-called" complication. Obtaining consent from a patient to publish may make you aware if a lawsuit is planned by the patient.

Although I concur with the requirement to get consent from the patient to publish case reports, it is a fact that it has become more and more difficult in the last 5 years to get case reports accepted by journals. This is most likely because journals are trying to obtain/maintain a high impact factor (citation rate). This has been highlighted by Mason [2]. He titled his editorial: "The case report – an endangered species." In it he talks about the impact factor (citation rate) and how it is calculated. It is worked out by: "dividing the total number of citations, received in any given year to articles published in the previous 2 years, by the total number of citable (or source) items." The term "source" in this case refers to original articles, reviews, and case reports, but not abstracts, editorials, or book reviews. The citation count includes all types of documents." It is the Institute for Scientific Information that does the citation analysis. Since case reports are rarely cited, it is obvious that journals who want a higher impact factor are no longer publishing as many case reports as previously. With less case reports, the journal will have a higher impact factor. Therefore, several journals like Anesthesia and Analgesia now have a separate journal dealing only with case reports. This may be seen as an encouraging development but, that said, few people read this publication.

Another reason for having difficulty in getting case reports accepted in journals is that the criteria of most, if not all, cases should involve only rare diseases (not seen before) or comorbidity (not described) and how they were dealt with. This is of very little interest to the clinician, who would generally prefer to read about problems occurring in his/her everyday practice and how to solve them or attempt to prevent them.

Lesson

1. Journals are accepting less and less case reports. Large journals have now established specialized sub-journals that deal purely with case reports. This is done so that the main journal's impact factor is not reduced.
2. Before a case report is accepted for review, journals now require a written consent from patients to publish their case.
3. If you have an interesting case, it is advisable to get the written consent as soon as you can, preferably before the patient leaves the hospital.

References

1. Hubregtse G, Collins SJ. Patient consent and case reports. Anaesthesia. 2001;56:906.
2. Mason RA. The case reports – an endangered species? Anaesthesia. 2001;56:99–102.

Chapter 57
Case 57: Are Case Reports Becoming Extinct?

As you read in Case 56, it has become harder and harder to get a case report published, unless it contains an account of a previously unpublished rare case with severe/uncommon comorbidities.

But if you had a case like the one below, would you think it would be worthwhile trying to get it published?

"The patient was an otherwise healthy 35-year-old (ASA1) undergoing a routing laparoscopic cholecystectomy. At the end of the case, before the endotracheal tube was removed, an oral gastric tube (OGT) was inserted but met resistance in the lower esophagus and was removed. The patient's head was repositioned and a new attempt was made. But again resistance was felt. As the OGT was removed bright red blood (60 mL) was seen coming from the OGT. An ENT surgeon was called but, when he arrives there was no more blood to be seen. The ENT surgeon correctly decides to do an esophagogastroduodenoscopy while the patient was still asleep. A mucosal tear was discovered at the end of the esophagus with no obvious sign of perforation or bleeding. Conservative management was recommended.

The patient was allowed to wake up and the trachea extubated. Thirty minutes later while in the recovery room, his oxygen saturation fell, despite oxygen 100 % being delivered by a non-rebreathing mask. A pneumothorax was diagnosed and a chest tube placed. In the ICU an esophagram showed an esophageal perforation."

The resident who has written the above draft understands that the case does not challenge doctrine and describe a rare event or even a rare disease, but he thinks it has an important teaching lesson.

What do you think? Should you attempt to submit it for publication?

© Springer Science+Business Media New York 2015

J.G. Brock-Utne, *Clinical Research*, DOI 10.1007/978-1-4939-2516-2_57

Answer/Solution

Submit for publication.

Discussion

Tim Angelotti [1] in an excellent editorial discusses the dilemma that researchers face in submitting and editors have in accepting for publication simple observations such as the one above [2]. As Dr. Angelotti so succinctly says: "One could easily understand how blood in an OG tube after removal, without subsequent re-bleeding, could be just dismissed as a minor trauma and ignored. If this type of thinking had been followed, the complication that occurred in the post-anesthesia care unit probably would have been missed, delaying care."

This is therefore a case report, not about a rare disease, a challenging case, etc., but about a common problem in an otherwise healthy patient. It informs you that you must be acutely aware of complications that can occur and how to prevent/deal with them.

Lesson

If you have a case that illustrates an important teaching point, always attempt to publish.

References

1. Angelotti T. (Editorial Comment): Esophageal perforation and pneumothorax after routine intraoperative orogastric tube placement. Anesth Analg (cases). 2014;2:125.
2. Turabi AA, Urton RJ, Anton TM, Herrmann R, Kwiatkowski D. Esophageal perforation and pneumothorax after routine intraoperative oro-gastric tube placement. Anesth Analg (cases). 2014;2:122–3.

Chapter 58
Case 58: A Clinical Pharmacology Study

A young researcher asks if you have any comments to make about a proposed study, which is summarized below:

The study is a double-blinded evaluation of two nonnarcotic drugs, each given in a single dose. The study is randomized, with a parallel-group design. The endpoint is morphine sparing. The surgical operations are all hysterectomies, in 45–75 years old.

What is your response?

© Springer Science+Business Media New York 2015   155
J.G. Brock-Utne, *Clinical Research*, DOI 10.1007/978-1-4939-2516-2_58

Answer/solution

To make a meaningful comparison between two drugs, one must compare dose–response relationships. This means that one must include at least two therapeutic effects. Obviously studying toxic doses is not considered ethical.

Discussion

A placebo should be included. By having a placebo, the study will show if the two drugs are analgesics. Let's say that the two drugs, in single doses, show no difference. Then does that mean that the two drugs are equally efficient in providing analgesia or does it mean that they are not effective as an analgesic? It is impossible to say without a placebo.

To do this study with a placebo and with one more dose of each drug, the researcher would need to increase the number of patients studied. The question would be: Are there enough patients in the hospital to have the study completed in a reasonable time frame? If not, then he will have to resort to a multicenter study.

Lesson

In a pharmacological study, it is important to have a dose–response study design, preferably with a placebo.

Chapter 59
Case 59: Watch Out

A visiting anesthesiologist, who was on sabbatical at our department, introduced us to a new monitoring equipment. We were all very excited. He had published his results in several journals. After reading his many papers, we could understand the need for more studies. We got IRB approval and completed a study with 60 patients. The methodology we used in our study was identical to his previous work. The results were interesting and worthy of publication, as they added more to the knowledge of this equipment. We all felt that the results could benefit patient care. We did not think there would be a problem in getting this work published.

We were surprised to learn that the paper was rejected, not by one but by several journals including two journals that had published the visitor's work earlier.

What would you do? Give up or what?

© Springer Science+Business Media New York 2015
J.G. Brock-Utne, *Clinical Research*, DOI 10.1007/978-1-4939-2516-2_59

Answer/Solution

Do a new literature search for this equipment.

Discussion

Unfortunately we learned that in the last year, considerable controversy about the equipment had surfaced. There were deep divisions in the medical community as to what the monitor actually measured.

Whenever you get involved with a research project, you must do a literature search. You need to know all there is to know about all the aspects of the proposed study. There are many online resources like Biosis, Cinahl, Cochrane Library (good for review articles), Embase, Google, Medline, PsycInfo, PubMed, Social Science Citation Index, and Web of Science. All these Web-based programs have become much more "user-friendly" since I started exploring them many years ago. It is still important to find the right key phrases and questions. If you don't find anything, modify your search and try again. If you still do not find anything, consider asking a searching professional. It is important to spend time on your search so that you don't miss anything.

Supino and Borer [1] state that a proper literature search should seek to answer the following questions:

1. Has the problem been previously addressed? If so, was it adequately studied? Are there any limitations to the study(s)? Have the researchers themselves identified limitations of their study?
2. Are the proposed hypotheses supported by current theory or knowledge?
3. Does the methodology cited in the literature provide guidance on available instrumentation for measuring variables?
4. Are the results of prior studies informative for calculation of sample size and power?
5. What are the conclusions drawn? Do you agree with them?
6. Did previous investigators suggest areas for future study? Has this been done by them or others?

In addition Supino and Borer [1] suggest creating an ongoing automatic search so that one is kept abreast of comparable research as it is published. I have found ResearchGate to be excellent in this way.

Lesson

1. If you get involved with a research project, you must check your facts. Know all there is to know about all the aspects of the proposed study.
2. If you are to use new equipment, make sure you know all there is to know about it and its limitations. If you don't, your research could prove to be a massive waste of time with no publication.

Reference

1. Supino PG, Borer JS. Principles of research methodology, A guide for clinical investigators. New York: Springer; 2012.

Chapter 60
Case 60: A New Equipment

A young resident shows you (an attending surgeon) a FDA-approved medical equipment which he has slightly altered so it can have a different function. Initially the resident wants to study it in volunteer. You decide that the altered equipment has a potentially beneficial function and should be totally harmless to the subjects.

The resident tells you he wants to study six volunteers with IRB approval. He wonders if you will be the first volunteer.

What is your response?

© Springer Science+Business Media New York 2015
J.G. Brock-Utne, *Clinical Research*, DOI 10.1007/978-1-4939-2516-2_60

Answer/Solution

While you do not want to hinder innovation, you should be opposed to sanctioning the improper use of any equipment. Hence, you should decline.

Discussion

When one alters the function of any equipment, one has in fact invented a new piece of equipment. The above resident could be viewed as a manufacturer, with all the medical legal responsibility that may follow. The use of any piece of equipment for any purpose other than that for which it was designed places both the producer of the device and its user in a potentially dangerous position.

In this case, it may be that the local IRB will approve the volunteer study. But should the results prove favorable, then one should not publish them until the FDA or similar institutions have approved the device for clinical use.

Lesson

Do not be unsympathetic to new ideas.

But always make sure that any research like the one proposed above is undertaken properly. That means the study must have an IRB approval and an appropriate investigational device permit obtained from the FDA.

Chapter 61
Case 61: Those That Ignore the Past

A visiting anesthesiologist demonstrates the superficial temporal arterial cannulation (STA) in infants. This he recommends instead of the radial artery (RA) cannulation. You are impressed, and under his guidance, you, as a resident, do one with great success. The visiting anesthesiologist suggests that you do ten cases, and if successful report it as an abstract to a pediatric medical meeting. He tells you he will help you with the IRB submission. You are excited.

However what should you do prior to starting this study?

© Springer Science+Business Media New York 2015
J.G. Brock-Utne, *Clinical Research*, DOI 10.1007/978-1-4939-2516-2_61

Answer/Solution

Do a literature review.

Discussion

You now find that there is a severe potentially lethal problem with this technique, and it should not be used on a routine basis [1, 2].

You will find Simmon's [3] article in particular worth reviewing. In it he and his colleagues attributed the STA cannulation to cause massive infarction in the distribution of the middle cerebral artery. It is of interest to note that the STA cannulation technique came to an abrupt halt after the publication of this article.

Armed with the literature review finding, you ask the visiting attendant about these complications. The reply from the attendant is that he has never seen it.

I know I have stressed previously in this book how important it is to review the literature before embarking on any clinical study. I do not apologize for repeating it again. This is especially true when you are contemplating doing a procedure which could potentially harm the patient.

Lesson

Always check your facts with a literature review and do not ignore past experiences.

References

1. Prian GW, Wright GB, Rumack CM, et al. Apparent cerebral embolization after temporal artery catheterization. J Pediatr. 1978;93:115–8.
2. Simmons MA, Levine RI, Lubchenco LO, et al. Warning: serious sequel of temporal artery catheterization. J Pediatr. 1978;92:284.
3. Baum VC. Those who ignore the past. Pediatr Anesth. 2007;18:191–2.

Chapter 62
Case 62: What Are the Safety Data for This Formulation?

You have just joined a department as an instructor. Several of the department's members are studying an FDA-approved drug that is being used intrathecally for which you don't think it is approved. You are asked to be involved.

You review the packet insert and see that it is recommended that the drug is not used in the intrathecal space. You are surprised that the study has been approved by the local IRB but note that in the application there is a mention of two published abstracts dealing with small human studies that show no bad outcomes.

Should you be involved or should you decline?

© Springer Science+Business Media New York 2015
J.G. Brock-Utne, *Clinical Research*, DOI 10.1007/978-1-4939-2516-2_62

Answer/Solution

This is an ethical dilemma that only you can answer.

Discussion

We were faced with this problem when we wanted to use ketamine intrathecally. Using monkeys and baboons, we examined their spinal nerve roots and were able to show that ketamine was safe [1, 2]. Human studies followed, but ketamine was found, in our study, to be short lasting [3]. However, others have used it with success [4].

If you are faced with this dilemma, you are strongly advised to read the editorials [5, 6] and papers dealing with intrathecal midazolam [7–9], both in sheep and humans. There are many clinical studies that have studied non-approved drugs in the intrathecal space [10]. These include, among others, sufentanil, meperidine, magnesium, sameridine, chloroprocaine, nalbuphine, and morphine-6-glucuronide [10]. It is worth reading the 2007 Anesthesia and Analgesia (A&A) Guide for Authors [11] and the article by Eisenach et al. [12]. As regards neuraxial administration the guide lines are as follows:

1. Is the drug approved by the FDA for this indication?
2. If the drug is not approved, is it widely used off-label (e.g., in tens of thousands of patients)? The A&A editorial board concluded that if multiple textbooks indicated that the drug could be safely used in a given manner, then that was a reasonable surrogate demonstration that the drug could be considered used for the indication.
3. If neither 1 nor 2 applies, was the study performed with an "Investigator Investigational New Drug (IND)" from the FDA or an equivalent regulatory authority?

Another ethical dilemma are studies involving FDA-approved drugs in larger than recommended doses [13] or the use of investigational drugs in humans [14–16]. The latter raises serious and valid concerns about the ethics of publishing a case report in which the use of an investigational drug has been used without prior informed consent even if it is an emergency.

Lesson

Before you or any patient gets involved with studies of this type, is it not fair to ask as Yaksh and Allen [6] says so eloquently: "And what are the safety data for this formulation?"

References

1. Brock-Utne JG, Mankowitz E, Kallichurum S, Downing JW. Effects of intrathecal saline and ketamine with or without preservatives on the spinal nerve roots of monkeys. S Afr Med J. 1982;61:360–1.
2. Brock-Utne JG, Kallichurum S, Mankowitz E, Maharaj RH, Downing JW. Intrathecal ketamine with preservative. Histological effects on the spinal nerve roots in baboons. S Afr Med J. 1982;61:440–1.
3. Mankowitz E, Brock-Utne JG, Cosnett JE, Green-Thompson R. Epidural ketamine. A preliminary report. S Afr Med J. 1982;61:441–2.
4. Congedo E, Sgreccia M, De Cosmo G. New drugs for epidural analgesia. Curr Drug Targets. 2009;10(8):696–706. Review.
5. Cousins MJ, Miller RD. Intrathecal midazolam: an ethical editorial dilemma. Anesth Analg. 2004;98:1507–8.
6. Yaksh TL, Allen JW. Preclinical insights into the implementation of intrathecal midazolam: a cautionary tale. Anesth Analg. 2004;98:1509–11.
7. Tucker AP, Lai C, Nadeson R, Goodchild CS. Intrathecal midazolam 1: a cohort study investigating safety. Anesth Analg. 2004;98:1512–20.
8. Tucker AP, Mezzatesta J, Nadeson R, Goodchild CS. Intrathecal midazolam 11: combination with intrathecal fentanyl for labor pain. Anesth Analg. 2004;98:1521–7.
9. Johansen MJ, Lee Gradert TL, Satterfield WC, Baze WB, Hildebrand K, Trissel L, Hassenbusch SJ. Safety of continuous intrathecal midazolam infusion in the sheep model. Anesth Analg. 2004;98:1528–35.
10. Shafer SL. Anesthesia & Analgesia's policy on off-label drug administration in clinical trials. Anesth Analg. 2007;105:13–5.
11. Anesthesia & Analgesia guide for authors. Anesth Analg. 2007;105:187–99.
12. Eishenach JC, James III FM, Gordh Jr T, Yaksh TL. New epidural drugs: primum non Nocere. Anesth Analg. 1998;87:1211–2.
13. Ramsay MAE, Luterman DL. Dexmedetomidine as a total intravenous anesthetic agent. Anesthesiology. 2004;101:787–90.
14. Lenz A, Hill G, White PF. The emergency use of sugammadex after failure of standard reversal drugs. Anesth Analg. 2007;104:585–6.
15. Rosman EJ. Pseudo-emergent use of an investigational drug. Anesth Analg. 2007;105:876.
16. Shafer SL. Pseudo-emergent use of an investigational drug. Anesth Analg. 2007;105:876.

Chapter 63
Case 63: This Is a Test to See What You Have Learned

You are listening to a presentation by a junior member of staff. He has just completed a study entitled:

"Isoflurane has a similar incidence of emergence agitation/delirium as sevoflurane in young children—a randomized controlled study."

The reason for the study is that many children become agitated or even delirious following general anesthesia, using volatile anesthetics. There are conflicting results from previous studies which compare two volatile anesthetics (isoflurane and sevoflurane) and the incidence of postoperative emergence agitation/delirium.

The study by the junior member is summarized.

Eighty children scheduled for inguinal hernia repair were included in the study. All were premedicated with oral midazolam. Anesthesia was induced either intravenously ($n=25$) or as an inhalational induction ($n=55$). After the children were asleep, they were randomized to receive either sevoflurane or isoflurane for anesthesia maintenance. After induction, a caudal was inserted for pain relief. No postoperative pain scores were presented.

The conclusion to this study was that there was no difference in the incidence of agitation (A) and/or delirium (D) between the two inhalational agents.

Now that you have read the many cases in this book, let's see if you have any good questions/concerns about the study design and its conclusions? There are at least seven.

© Springer Science+Business Media New York 2015
J.G. Brock-Utne, *Clinical Research*, DOI 10.1007/978-1-4939-2516-2_63

Answer/Solution

There are several questions you should consider:

1. Was a power analysis done prior to the start of the study?
2. What was the difference in A/D between the children who got an intravenous induction and the ones who got an inhalational induction? Why not exclude the group who got the intravenous induction?
3. Premedication with midazolam has been shown to decrease the incidence of delirium. Is it possible that midazolam is more effective in preventing A/D when isoflurane is used as compared to sevoflurane?
4. The intravenous agent, thiopentone, has been associated with decreased A/D.
5. What scale was used to assess the agitation/delirium? Has the scale been validated in previous similar studies? How were the assessors trained in the use of this scale?
6. Were the parents present during the induction of anesthesia in all cases or only some? If the parents were not present during the induction, were there any measurement done to judge separation anxiety? Did the score vary from the isoflurane to the sevoflurane group?
7. How effective was the pain relief? What were the postoperative pain scores? Any difference between the groups?

Despite the questions/concerns raised following the presentation, our young colleague submitted the paper for publication. As can be expected, the manuscript was not accepted. The editor and reviewers found the title misleading, had many of the above concerns, and concluded that the paper added very little to our knowledge of this problem.

Lesson

There are so many factors that contribute to a clinical research outcome. Make sure you make the study simple, have enough power, and don't include subgroups with different methodologies. If you are using a clinical scale to evaluate A/D, it is imperative to make sure it has been validated in the group you are studying and that the coworkers doing the testing have been adequately trained.

Appendix A
Review of the Clinical Research Process.
From the Beginning to the End

1. Identify the clinical research question.
2. Consider all aspects that may stand in your way in completing the proposed study like

   (a) Have you enough patients?
   (b) Can the study be done within 12 months?
   (c) Have you got all the equipment and help you need?

3. Obtain IRB approval.
4. If the study involves using patients who are also seen by other departments, then it is imperative that those departments' members are informed about the study and maybe involve them as authors.
5. Decide on who the authors will be and the order in which they should appear in the manuscript.
6. When the study is finished, write an abstract that can be submitted to your annual society meeting. If various departments are participating, then abstracts can be submitted to various annual society meetings. Presenting at meetings can give you valuable feedback, before you write the final version of your paper.
7. Decide to which journal you want to submit it to.
8. Read the instructions for authors AGAIN and follow them.
9. Write the first draft, with working title, and design tables/figures with titles and footnotes/legends.
10. Apply for permission to reproduce any previously published tables, figures, or other material that will be used.
11. Check completeness of the references and follow the journals instructions on how to write your references.
12. Send the draft to your coworkers for their comments. It is very important to put a time limit on their response. I usually say within 48 h.
13. Make any necessary alterations.

© Springer Science+Business Media New York 2015
J.G. Brock-Utne, *Clinical Research*, DOI 10.1007/978-1-4939-2516-2

14. Decide on a title and the final order of authors.
15. Obtain a critical review from a senior colleague if possible.
16. Write your cover letter to the editor, giving permission to reproduce any published material or to cite unpublished work.
17. Make sure that all photographs, etc., are included in the submission and keep copies of everything. Don't send the only photos you have.
18. Send the final copy to all authors.
19. The cover letter should summarize what is included in the submission.
20. If the paper is to be published, accept all suggestions gracefully. Obviously if you strongly disagree with a specific suggestion/comment, you should respectfully argue your case.
21. Correct the galley proofs in a timely fashion. If you can't do it, get your coworkers to do it.
22. If the editor rejects the paper, revise it as necessary, even the title, and send it elsewhere, or put it in your drawer.

Appendix B
The Future of Clinical Research

It is difficult to predict the future path for clinical research. Most likely, we will need more studies that compare animal and human responses to address basic mechanisms for clinical questions. This may certainly be true in neuroscience. For example, a study by MacIver et al. [1] paves the way for such an approach. They used microelectrode recordings from human neurons and from similar neurons in rat brain slices. Electrophysiologic events were analyzed before and after administration of either propofol or remifentanil. Neither drug produced major alterations of subthalamic neuron discharge activity, although the changes seen in humans were readily explained by drug actions seen at the synaptic level in brain slice recordings. Findings from this study showed that both of these agents could be used during the mapping phase of electrode implant surgery to relieve patient anxiety and facilitate comfort and safety.

One thing is sure and that is that our future standard of medical care will be only as good as the clinical trials we subject the various techniques, equipment, and drugs to. The long-term survival of clinical research will be based on our contribution to patient's improved health. As physicians we are observant and practical [2]. We recognize problems that matter and should, with clinical research, implement solutions that work, based on verifiable evidence.

References

1. MacIver MB, Bronte-Stewart HM, Henderson JM, Jaffe RA, Brock-Utne JG. Human subthalamic neuron spiking exhibits subtle responses to sedatives. Anesthesiology. 2011;115:254–64.
2. Shorten GD. Anaesthesia, research and translation: "…send not to know for whom the Bell tolls…" (Editorial). Anaestheia. 2007;62:211–3.

Appendix C
Summary Pearls

1. Run the research as a business. Be efficient, not tardy. Deliver on time. If you are doing a sponsored study, say that you hope to be finished by December 15, but in actual fact you plan to deliver the final results on October 15.
2. Don't pressure/require anyone to do clinical research. This is, in my experience, doomed to failure. As they say: "You can take a horse to water, but you can't make it drink."
3. You don't do research to become famous or wealthy, especially at the expense of others.
4. Make sure you are using the appropriate statistics. For example, when comparing two monitors, don't do a linear regression analysis but a Bland–Altman plot (Lancet 1985, i:307–10). The latter plots the differences versus the average of the monitors on a scatter plot. The plot will tell you how reliable a new measurement is.

As an El Toro clinical researcher, you may find the task ahead daunting. Remember that you do not have to be a statistician, epidemiologist, mathematician, engineer, or a computer scientist, etc.; the only thing that is required is for you to have important questions, a great passion to achieve, and surround yourself with people who can do all the other stuff.

Good luck and have fun.

John G. Brock-Utne, M.D., Ph.D.

© Springer Science+Business Media New York 2015
J.G. Brock-Utne, *Clinical Research*, DOI 10.1007/978-1-4939-2516-2

Index

Printed in the United States
By Bookmasters